Brent Q. Hafen is a professor of health sciences at Brigham Young University and the co-author of many best-selling books, most recently *How to Live Longer* and *Emotional Survival* (Prentice-Hall).

Kathryn J. Frandsen is a press secretary in Washington, D.C. Formerly, she was an editor at Brigham Young University Press and a writer/editor for a major advertising agency.

PRENTICE-HALL INTERNATIONAL, INC., London
PRENTICE-HALL OF AUSTRALIA PTY. LIMITED, Sydney
PRENTICE-HALL CANADA INC., Toronto
PRENTICE-HALL OF INDIA PRIVATE LIMITED, New Delhi
PRENTICE-HALL OF JAPAN, INC., Tokyo
PRENTICE-HALL OF SOUTHEAST ASIA PTE. LTD., Singapore
WHITEHALL BOOKS LIMITED, Wellington, New Zealand
EDITORA PRENTICE-HALL DO BRASIL LTDA., Rio de Janeiro

FROM ACUPUNCTURE TO YOGA

Alternative Methods of Healing

BRENT Q. HAFEN
KATHRYN J. FRANDSEN

A SPECTRUM BOOK

Prentice-Hall, Inc., Englewood Cliffs, New Jersey 07632

Library of Congress Cataloging in Publication Data

Hafen, Brent Q.
  From acupuncture to yoga.

  "A Spectrum Book"—Verso t.p.
  Includes bibliographical references and index.
    1. Therapeutics, Physiological.   2. Healing.
  I. Frandsen, Kathryn J.   II. Title.   [DNLM: 1. Medicine,
  Traditional.   2. Holistic health.   3. Therapeutic
  cults.   WB 890 H138f]
  RM700.H33 1983   615.8   82-24008
  ISBN 0-13-330845-6
  ISBN 0-13-330837-5 (pbk.)

CONTENTS

PREFACE

You have probably heard of some of the alternative healing methods, and you have probably been curious about what you have heard. Maybe you have dabbled in a few techniques, and maybe you have been firmly convinced one way or another.

These alternatives are the unconventional approaches to healing and health. Some have gained widespread acceptance and approval from the orthodox medical community: osteopathic medicine is one such practice. But many others are still viewed with suspicion and sometimes with outright hostility. Their claims remain unsubstantiated, while hundreds of thousands of advocates continue to practice the principles that lie behind them.

This volume is intended simply to explain the principles of the various philosophies of health and healing. It is not intended to endorse, nor is it intended to condemn. Its purpose is to educate consumers about the variety of approaches taken, both in orthodox and unorthodox medicine, in the complex job of healing those who are ill.

Some of the alternative methods discussed here are presented merely as philosophies, whereas other methods are presented as philosophies combined with techniques. We present some methods merely as philosophies because to perform these methods of healing, special instruction or education is required. It is not within the scope of this book to introduce such material. On the other hand, many of the methods are presented with accompanying techniques. In some cases you may be able, from the explanation given, to experiment with some of these alternative forms of treatment for relief of minor complaints.

Please use extreme caution! Although this volume neither endorses nor condemns any of the practices discussed, we strongly urge you not to attempt self-treatment after reading a certain therapy—even though you may feel convinced that you are well enough informed from the material presented in this book. If you are interested in any of the therapies discussed in this volume, you should contact practitioners or instructors who can counsel and supervise you in your attempts at practicing any of the therapies.

Please exercise extreme caution, too, in seeking treatment for serious or life-threatening conditions. Under no circumstances should you attempt self-treatment for a serious condition; seek help from a reputable health professional who can direct you to treatment alternatives.

THE CONCEPT
OF
HOLISTIC HEALTH

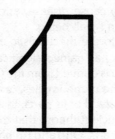

Traditionally, medicine has been mechanistic: doctors and other health-care specialists have pictured the body as a machine, with separate parts that must be treated separately.[1] The mechanistic approach to medicine stresses the physician's role in treating disease, downplays the mental and emotional factors that may cause disease, and ignores completely the spiritual aspect of health and well-being.

In sharp contrast to the mechanistic approach is an approach termed *holistic health* that has gained significant momentum since its recent introduction. *Holistic* is derived from the Greek word *holos*, meaning "whole." Holism, as the name implies, is a philosophy that entails treating the whole body, instead of its parts, in a total environment. This concept comes from the ancient theory that the universe and all living nature are the sum of their parts. Otto and Knight define holistic health as "the treatment of the whole person. It helps to bring the mental/emotional, physical, social, spiritual dimensions of the person's being into harmony and employs wholistic principles and the elements of a total, integrated treatment program, with emphasis on any therapy or treatment that stimulates a person's own healing processes."[2] Holistic health is seen as a wholeness, a balanced and harmonious function of the body, the mind, and the spirit—the spirit being that force which gives meaning and direction to life and provides a sense of inner happiness.

The holistic health philosophy of medicine stands in stark con-

2

trast to mechanistic health because it acknowledges the importance of the spiritual element of health; the mental and emotional factors in well-being and disease are recognized and treated.

Holism goes further, however, in stressing the individual's responsibility for maintaining good health—a personal responsibility that includes recognition of the physical, mental, emotional, and spiritual components that make up the whole. By working with the individual and emphasizing the self-responsibility for health, holism provides an encouragement that helps to prevent disease and emphasizes wellness. Thus, the individual becomes a self-healer in a sense and an active partner in health care, rather than a passive recipient.

The holistic philosophy has been influential for thousands of years. One of the best-known practitioners of our times was mystic Edgar Cayce, born more than 100 years ago in Hopkinsville, Kentucky.[3] His technique was to enter sleep trances in which he dictated his philosophies of life and healing, and he was widely recognized as a healer until his death in 1944. The Cayce Foundation still operates in Virginia Beach, Virginia. Cayce's alternative methods of healing, and other holistic methods like them, spread rapidly to the west coast, and a number of academies, foundations, and associations currently operate across the country.[4]

In practice, holistic health includes all health-promoting approaches. According to Michael Halberstam, "Holistic health, by definition, is all-embracing."[5] Holism is medically and morally neutral. Holistic health seeks to understand all systems without getting locked into any of them. It complements and encompasses whatever system, method, or means best promotes optimum health. Figure 1 illustrates some of the approaches that are included in holistic health.

The holistic approach extends to the prevention of disease, maintenance of good health, and healing of disease.[6] Traditional medicine is centered around the theory that certain bacteria and viruses lead to infection and disease, and traditional healing regimens have concentrated on using medication to halt disease. Little prevention is involved. The holistic approach, on the other hand, maintains that weakened resistance—brought about by poor habits and physical and mental stress—makes the body susceptible to disease. Disease is seen as the result of an imbalance among a variety of social, personal, and economic, as well as biologic, influences.[7] Paavo O. Airola, a leading

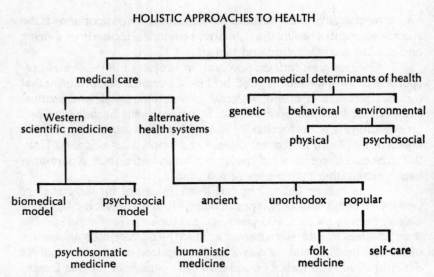

HOLISTIC APPROACHES TO HEALTH

Figure 1 (From David S. Sobel, *Ways of Health* edited and copyright (c) 1979 by David S. Sobel. Reprinted by permission of Harcourt Brace Janovich, Inc.)

exponent of holistic health and healing, identified those stresses and influences as tensions, fears, worries, and other emotional stresses; exogenous poisons from polluted water, air, and food; toxic drugs, tobacco, and alcohol; poor nutritional patterns, such as overeating, excessive protein intake, too much refined sugar, overindulgence in fats, and consequent retention of metabolic wastes; and lack of sufficient exercise, rest, and relaxation.[8]

The holistic approach, then, is centered on prevention and is a method of restoring a balance within the individual and between the individual and the environment.

On the basis of this concept of disease, proponents of holistic health have formulated the following basic principles for healing.

1. Every human being has vast untapped potentials, resources, and powers that can be used to further the process of holistic healing.
2. Self-awareness and understanding can enhance the healing process.
3. To mobilize the healing process, all the capabilities, resources, and talents of the individual should be used and tapped.

4

4. The importance of the patient and his relationship to the environment should be recognized.
5. The self-regulating processes should be used to control the disease state before the physical manifestations of the disease show up.
6. Group interaction can play a big part in holistic healing.
7. Bringing increased harmony to life can aid the healing process.
8. The individual's personal belief structure should be considered when choosing a healing method. While some healing methods do not rely on the patient's faith in the treatment, other healing systems are partially dependent on personal beliefs of the patient.[9]

In addition, holistic health takes into account the patient's genetic, biological, and psychosocial uniqueness so that the treatment prescribed for the patient meets his or her specific needs. Holistic health also seeks to understand and treat people in the context of culture, family, and community and emphasizes helping people to understand and help themselves, so the focus is on education and self-care rather than treatment and dependence. Diagnostic methods other than standard laboratory exams are used, and there is physical contact between the practitioner and the patient.

Illness becomes an opportunity for personal discovery, not just a time of misfortune. Thus, there is an appreciation of the quality of life in every state of health and an interest in improving it as well as dealing with major and minor illnesses.

Holistic health goes far beyond healing, in the sense that it strives to promote complete wellness or positive wellness. Proponents explain that complete wellness is more than just the absence of disease: it is a state of complete personal fulfillment and harmony. Some of the concomitant benefits may include vitality and enthusiasm about life; joyful life experiences; trimness and physical fitness; freedom from minor complaints and health-destroying habits; alertness, clear-headedness and ability to concentrate; adequate sleep and nutrition; freedom from anxiety and worry; self-assuredness, self-assertion, confidence, and optimism; satisfaction with work as meaningful and productive; satisfaction with the direction of life; sexual fulfillment with profound love relationships; fulfillment and peace with the inner self; valuable contributions to the lives of others; and minimal tension and stress.[10]

PREVENTION

Of primary importance to proponents of holistic health is prevention, taking necessary steps to maintain health at a level that enables prevention of disease initially. In a speech introducing the controversial Hospital Cost Containment Act, former President Jimmy Carter stressed that "Prevention is both cheaper and simpler than cure."[11] Despite our strides in medical research, he said, fourteen nations have lower infant mortality rates than that of the United States; as recently as 1974, 47 percent of all United States children under the age of five had not been immunized against polio, 44 percent had not been immunized against rubella, and 40 percent were not protected from measles. Thousands of women die from cervical and uterine cancer each year,[12] yet the Pap test, devised in 1943 as a measure to detect those cancers, is a painless test that is inexpensive and easy to perform. As recently as 1974, one-fourth of the nation's women had *never* had a Pap test.

With a shift of emphasis to prevention of disease, claim the proponents of holistic health, individuals would take full responsibility for maintaining their own health—including a responsibility to prevent the onset of disease by altering environmental and lifestyle factors that might lead to the development of disease.

NOTES

1. Harold H. Bloomfield. "Holistic: The New Reality in Health," *New Realities,* April 1977, p. 9.
2. Herbert A. Otto and James W. Knight, "Wholistic Healing: Basic Principles and Concepts," in Herbert A. Otto and James W. Knight, eds. *Dimensions in Wholistic Healing: New Frontiers in the Treatment of the Whole Person.* Nelson-Hall: Chicago, 1979, p. 4.
3. John P. Callan. "Holistic Health or Holistic Hoax," *Journal of the American Medical Association*, March 16, 1979, p. 1156.
4. Ibid.
5. Michael Halberstam. "Holistic Healing: Limits of 'the New Medicine'" *Psychology Today*, August 1978, p. 26.
6. Paavo O. Airola. "The Holistic Approach to Total Health," *New Realities*, April 1979, p. 17.

7. Milton Friedman. "Holistic Health: Is Washington Listening?" *New Realities*, April 1979, p. 19.

8. Airola, p. 18.

9. Otto and Knight, pp. 8-11.

10. C. Norman Shealy. "Holistic Management of Chronic Pain and Distress," *New Realities*, April 1979, p. 68; Bloomfield, p. 15.

11. Jimmy Carter, "Preventive Health Care," in Edward Bauman, et al, eds. *The Holistic Health Handbook*. And/Or Press: Berkeley, California, 1978, p. 20.

12. Carter, p. 30.

FROM ORIENTAL TO AMERICAN INDIAN: MAJOR COMPREHENSIVE SYSTEMS

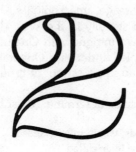

ORIENTAL MEDICINE

Public interest in various aspects of Oriental medicine—including acupuncture, shiatsu massage, macrobiotics, herbal medicine, and moxibustion—has grown steadily in the West during the past several decades. Although Western intrigue with Oriental medicine is a recent phenomenon, the principles underlying Oriental medicine are ancient and have their base in Taoism, a school of thought that dates back to prehistoric times.

Five major principles determine Taoist belief:

- All phenomena exist within infinite space.
- All phenomena are interrelated.
- All phenomena are relative.
- Everything has energy or vibration.
- Everything is in a constant state of change.[1]

Taoists claim that there is constant movement between two poles: the yin and the yang, and that the energy (or vibration) between these two opposing poles is the activating force of all phenomena. They maintain that this constant flux, or movement, can be observed in all things—from the smallest molecule to the largest planet, throughout the entire universe.

The easiest way to understand the concept of yin and yang is to conceptualize yin as the tendency toward expansion (or centrifugality) and yang as the tendency toward contraction (or centripetality). According to the ancient Chinese, yin and yang are characterized by such qualities as:

Yin	Yang
Negative	Positive
Female	Male
Passive	Active
Earth	Sky
Moon	Sun
Plain	Splendid
Soft	Hard
Right	Left
White	Black
Even	Odd
Dark	Light
Cold	Warm
Emptiness	Fullness[2]

Because yin and yang are complementary forces, they must be in balance to create health in an individual or correct and optimal conditions in the universe.

The dynamic, subtle energy in all things, the vehicle through which the yin and yang operate, was called *ki* in Japan, *ch'i* in China, and *prana* in India. Everything—animal, vegetable, mineral, and human—has ki to some extent, according to this philosophy, but the energy level and the quality and rate of vibration differ in each. The food and drink we consume each day provide us with ki, and the goal of Oriental medicine is to regulate the intake of food and drink to maximize the harmonious flow of ki in the body.[3]

Proponents of this medicine group the body organs into pairs, each pair made up of a yin organ (a hollow organ of absorption, such as the gall bladder, or of discharge, such as the urinary bladder) and a yang organ (a dense, blood-filled organ of regulation, such as the heart or kidney) that have a complementary relationship. The ki level—or energy level—required to nourish each organ differs according to its density and structure. The various organs are classified as follows:

Yin (hollow)	Yang (compact)
Large intestine	Lungs
Gall bladder	Liver
Stomach	Spleen/pancreas
Urinary bladder	Kidney
Small intestine	Heart[4]

NATIVE AMERICAN HEALING

In the traditions of most of the Native American Indian tribes of this continent, healing practices are based on the belief that all healing is related to Mother Earth. Native Americans feel that everything on earth contains a spirit, and that the earth itself is a living, breathing organism capable of sensation. "The forces of all creation are dynamically interwoven into a harmonious whole,"[5] according to Sandy Newhouse and John Amodeo. Man, every phase of nature, the Earth, and the waters are a whole. Illness occurs when this balance and harmony between man and his environment are upset. Conversely, health is attained when man is living in a sensible, respectful relationship with the Earth and the environment.

Most Native American healing practices use music, dance, prayer, and ceremony to establish a relationship between man and Earth so that man can derive Earth's energy for healing purposes. These healing practices are also used to placate the evil powers responsible for illness and to attract the goodness which will re-establish the basic harmony between man and Earth that promotes the cure for illness. In addition, the healing practices serve to unite the individual to his deeper self to reestablish whatever harmony has been lost.

Ceremony is the expression of Indian life and healing, and all healing ceremonies center on the drum, which has a dual symbolism: the round shape is symbolic of the shape of the Earth, and the beat represents the heartbeat of everyone on Earth. Chants and songs are a vital part of the ceremony which unite the individual needing the healing, the medicine man, and the rest of the Indian community to accomplish the desired purpose.

A ceremony called Blessingway forms the framework of the ceremonial system among some Native American tribes. Blessingway can last as long as a month, but it is most commonly a two-day ceremony. Its duration is determined by the nature of the illness. It has three ceremonial divisions:

- Holyway, which attracts good spirits to cure and repair malfunctions.
- Evilway, which banishes the effects of evil things.
- Lifeway, which is responsible for curing physical illness and accidents.

During the performance of these ceremonies, the Indian community is united so that a communal effort is enacted on behalf of the sick. This unity has a strong psychosocial effect, and it may be one of the factors that effects healing.

A variety of techniques is utilized in American Indian healing ceremonies. One common pattern involves:

1. *Purification.* During purification, the patient and the medicine man are cleansed from any evil or malignant influences. This promotes an empty condition which makes them both receptive to healing energies and influences. The purification can be accomplished by fasting, sweating, emesis, sexual continence, bathing, shampooing the hair, and vigil.
2. *Evocation.* Evocation employs the invocatory rituals that invite the presence of the good and healing spirits. These rituals consist mainly of song sequences and sand paintings. It is thought that as sand paintings are created and subsequently blessed, the gods enter into the paintings to effect the healing.
3. *Identification.* During this phase of the ceremony, the patient is brought into psychic union with the powers that heal.
4. *Transformation.* During the transformation, the individual is freed from disease and disharmony. Both identification and transformation are accompanied by songs, prayers, and rites on the sand paintings.

5. *Release.* After a cure has been effected, the powers that have made the healing possible are disbursed.[6]

Medicine Men

The medicine man is one of the carriers of the culture and sometimes serves as spokesman for the group. Medicine men—and medicine women—are thought to have special electromagnetic vibrations that can effect healing by balancing the energy within the sick person.

The medicine man studies, meditates, and works at his practice from his earliest years. He could be said to be one of the earliest psychotherapists because part of the efficacy of his treatments and cures lies in the psychological realm. He often employs elaborate regalia and repetitious singing rituals to create a mood that promotes the desired psychological effects.

Ceremonial Adjuncts

In addition to his roles as physician and priest, the medicine man is generally a herbalist because plants are an important part of Native American healing. He is often in charge of the ceremonial garden and the preparation of plants for the ceremonies. Special care must be taken in growing and harvesting plants to be used ceremonially because of their great power. For example, before uprooting a ceremonial plant, the harvester must bring himself into harmony with the spirit of the plant so the healing power will not be destroyed.

Plants were commonly believed to have varying specific energies and healing powers. Many of the herbs and plants used in native American healing are distasteful, because their foul taste is thought to be injurious to the spirits causing the disease. Cedar, sage, and sweetgrass are often used in the purification part of the ceremony.

Prayer is another vital part of most American Indian healing ceremonies. Through prayer, vibrations from natural objects and activities can be attuned to the larger vibrations of the Earth and the Universe.

Two of the most popular means of curing are crystals and color healing. It is thought that quartz crystals have an electromagnetic energy similar to that of the human body and that a quartz crystal placed close to the body draws out any energy imbalance. Color healing is based upon the law of attraction: the vibrations of the color are believed to attract similar vibrations in the human body and to draw out the vibrations causing energy imbalance. Three color groups are used in color healing: the hot colors (red, orange, and yellow), the cool colors (blue, indigo, and violet), and green (the balance color). Specific colors are indicated for healing specific conditions.[7]

HOMEOPATHY

Homeopathic diagnosis and therapy also treats the whole body as a unified organism. Its basic tenets date to the early nineteenth century, when Samuel Friedrich Christian Hahnemann, its discoverer, defined disease itself as a nonentity and characterized it as "an aberration from the state of health" which cannot be mechanically removed from the body.[8] At the time, medical science relied on purging disease from the body with methods like "cupping," but Hahnemann concentrated on developing remedies like our medications of today. ("Cupping" is a procedure which makes use of metal or glass cups, or even a machine. Cotton wool, which has been soaked in alcohol or herbs, is placed inside the cup and burned. When the edges are cool enough, the cup is turned upside down and placed tightly against the skin. Inside the cup a vacuum is thus developed, creating suction and pulling the skin into the cup. Therapists use cupping for the following conditions: arthritic conditions, asthma, boils, bronchitis, painful congestion, pleurisy, pneumonia, and rheumatism. Some therapists apply the cupping technique in treating migraine headaches in conjunction with an acupuncture needle.)

The principles of homeopathic medicine, as laid down by Hahnemann in 1811, call for healing by the quickest, most reliable, and most permanent means available to the physician. Disease was considered to be of two types: *acute* conditions, which temporarily disable the body but may be overcome with treatment and time, and *chronic* conditions, a series of acute episodes that can, over time, seriously disable the body.

In treating either acute or chronic disabilities, the homeopathic physician is charged with four responsibilities: (1) a thorough knowledge of disease, including bacteriology, etiology, pathology, prognosis, and diagnosis; (2) a thorough acquaintance with the medicinal power of drugs; (3) an ability to relate the medicinal power of a drug to an individual patient's condition; and (4) an ability to foresee barriers between the patient and good health and a knowledge of how to reduce such barriers (which can include abstract entities like attitude and spiritual value deterioration).[9] Once the homeopathic physician has diagnosed the disease, he resorts to his repertory of medications and concocts a drug of sufficient potency to alleviate it. All of the remedies are derived from animal, vegetable, and mineral sources found in nature.

The treatment prescribed by the homeopathic physician is based on the idea that the body contains a vital, natural force which has the power to effect recovery and which reacts to stimulation from without. This vital force drives the human being and integrates the body, soul, and mind. Homeopathic treatments and remedies are designed to work on the level of this vital energy force.[10] The number of diseases in the world is infinite, so there is an infinite number of remedies.

Homeopathic treatments are based on four basic principles:

1. *The Law of Similars.* Samuel Hahnemann found that the bark of the cinchona tree alleviated the symptoms of malaria, but he found that in doing so, the bark produced symptoms very like the symptoms of malaria itself. This discovery led to the concept that "like cures like."[11] In other words, a drug which produces symptoms of a disease in a healthy person will cure a person who has the disease. In Hahnemann's words,

   Since the body's reactive force endeavors to cope with a given stress by producing a particular set of symptoms, the physician's duty is to promote the development of this very set of symptoms.[12]

   Homeopathy holds that when the patient receives the one remedy whose symptomatology most perfectly matches his or her own symptoms, the whole disease is removed, root and branch.[13]

   Only unhealthy cells or tissues will respond to the remedies, so few side effects are produced. Homeopathy proponents believe that killing the germ does not necessarily eliminate the disease cause, because the real underlying cause is the preexisting health state of the patient which enabled the disease to enter and multiply.

2. *The Law of Potentiation.* This law maintains that high doses of medicine intensify the symptoms of disease, whereas minute doses of medication tend to strengthen the body's defense mechanisms. Hence, the cure lies not in the quantity of medication taken but in the quality and subtle aspects of the curative treatment. Consequently, homeopathic medications are subjected to dilution, forceful shaking, and mixing. "The result of this process is a medicinal substance whose properties are extremely potent, yet nontoxic, as there is very little physical substance to cause toxicity."[14]

Homeopathic medications are prepared by soaking the remedial substance in a mixture of alcohol and water to make a tincture. One part of the tincture is then added to 99 parts alcohol and water and shaken vigorously. The resulting medicine has a potency that is termed 1. A medicine with a potency of 2 is made by adding one part of the potency 1 medicine to 99 parts ethyl alcohol and water and shaking vigorously. The alcohol-water ratio is based on multiples of 10: for example, 10:1 (ten parts alcohol); 100:1; 1000:1. Medications may be diluted repeatedly until their potency is vastly reduced.

3. *The Law of Cure.* The Law of Cure is stated as follows: A cure is effected "from above downwards; from within outwards; from a more important organ to a less important one; in reverse order of appearance"[15] of symptoms.

4. *Single Remedy.* The homeopath's medication consists of one pure drug at a time—never a mixture that might contain many chemical compounds.

NATUROPATHY

Naturopathy—meaning, literally, *nature cure*—originates from the time when man was a fully instinctive creature, and it embraces all the therapeutic methods that will guide the human organism back to its "original state of wholeness."[16]

According to proponents of naturopathy, there is a healing power present in all living things. Advocates claim that the natural tendency of all the cells in the body is to work toward the good of the whole body, which in turn works to maintain the good cells and to reject waste products.[17]

Naturopathy uses nature's agencies, forces, and products in concert with the inherent, natural healing power of the human body to effect cures. In seeking out natural products for a cure or therapy, naturopaths subscribe to a way of life which expands their awareness of nature and energy processes and achieve an environmental harmony, similar to the animals. This enables practitioners to lead and maintain a healthy life.

When disease is present, say naturopaths, the vital energy force and inherent healing powers are blocked. The goal of therapy, then, is to restore life force and the self-healing and balancing powers by natural means; for example, by removing toxic waste products resulting from either disease or normal metabolism, by restoring tissue vitality, and by reintegrating the body with the psychosocial element.

The naturopath does not use external therapeutics, such as surgery or drugs, to effect treatment, but instead commonly uses methods like fasting, hydrotherapy, massage, vitamin and mineral therapy, vegetarian diets, "health" foods, herbs, mud packs, joint manipulation, exercise, and colonic irrigation. Naturopaths may also use some of the methods employed by homeopaths and osteopaths.[18]

Unlike many healing systems, naturopathy does not concentrate on symptoms and cures, but on causes for the disease or its symptoms. The goal of therapy is to reverse or eliminate the causes by bringing the *whole* person into treatment. To eliminate disease and produce a condition of health, naturopaths generally rely on a combination of treatments rather than a single method; the naturopath may integrate diet, massage, hydrotherapy, and joint manipulation, for example.

Once viewed with skepticism, naturopathic medicine is now becoming more widely accepted. Students at naturopathic colleges are taught most of the same courses as students at orthodox medical schools, and naturopathic physicians practice in the same clinical areas as orthodox general practitioners—including pediatrics, geriatrics, gastroenterology, pulmonary disease, cardiology, neurology, and so on.

But there is a major difference in naturopathic medicine: the naturopath concentrates as much on preventing disease as he does on curing it. An orthodox general practitioner does not generally take time with patients to teach nutrition, exercise, and other preventive techniques; the naturopath integrates them as part of his medical practice. Most practitioners also include psychological counseling and therapy along with physical treatment and education on disease prevention.

Despite greater acceptance of naturopathic medicine, the legal status of the naturopath varies widely from one state to another: in some states the practice is totally prohibited, while other states openly license and regulate naturopaths. Some states allow them to practice under common law as long as they do not use drugs of any kind. Despite restrictions, there are naturopaths practicing in almost every state of the country.

ANTHROPOSOPHICAL MEDICINE

The theory of anthroposophical medicine was proposed by Rudolf Steiner, who intended the theory to be an extension of mainstream Western medicine, not an alternative to it.

Steiner saw reality as divided into two parts: sense perception and concept, or thought. He felt that man has to bring the two together by his own inner activity to get in touch with reality.

The theory behind anthroposophical medicine envisions the healthy human organism as a combination of three elements:

- A system of nerves and senses that provides a physical basis for sense perception and thinking.
- A system of metabolism and limbs that provides the physiological basis for the life of the will.
- A rhythmic system of circulation and respiration that is the basis of the life of feeling.

Anthroposophical thought holds that the fundamental basis for disease and illness is expressed in the idea that the body has two poles. The cool pole symbolizes the forces that are at rest, and it is represented by brain and nerve cells that are constantly dying. The warm pole represents movement, and it is symbolized by the metabolic cells which are always active in their capacity to regenerate. Consciousness is seen as arising from the continuous death process of the nerve cells.

Illness is seen as the process by which the individual can achieve greater freedom and wholeness. Proponents of anthroposophical medicine believe that a physician should not eliminate illness from the body or mind but merely guide it in the most beneficial way, since it ultimately helps the individual to become a more unified being.

Thus, remedies are given which do not destroy the disease process but merely aid the process in its completion and resolution. Steiner advocated remedies derived from minerals, plants, and animals.[19]

ASTROLOGY/MEDICAL ASTROLOGY

Astrology has been an adjunct to medicine and science for centuries. It is a practice that involves the study of planetary cycles, climacteric periods, and critical days, in conjunction with the time, date, and location of birth, to indicate the diseases to which a person may be susceptible. Proponents suggest that there is a correspondence between planetary patterns and specific diseases: some rhythms of the cosmic periods—that is, the signs of the zodiac, the houses of the horoscope, and the aspects between the planets—relate to certain illness conditions. These cosmic rhythms are similar to the circadian rhythms discussed in the section on biorhythms (see Chapter 6).

Although the sciences of medicine and astrology were inseparable in the ancient world, modern medical astrology is a fairly recent revival of that discredited subject. The practice now uses a correlation of patients' problems, both physical and mental, with their astrological charts to find the possible solution and prognosis of a condition, whether it is a crisis of body or soul. This therapeutic approach employs a theory of harmonics to diagnose problems and find a way to reunite body and soul.

Medical astrology can help the patient by:

1. Giving a general evaluation of strong and weak points; past, present, and potential problems; and present or potential illnesses.
2. Diagnosing disease conditions of the body and mind.

3. Guiding treatment by helping in appropriate therapy selection.
4. Clarifying the prognosis by projecting the problem into the future so that the patient can know the outcome of the condition and the optimum timing for therapy.
5. Giving information on the past, present, and future to help an individual formulate a health plan for life.[20]

NOTES

1. William Tara, "Oriental Medicine," in Ann Hill, ed. *A Visual Encyclopedia of Unconventional Medicine.* Crown Publishers Inc.: New York, 1979, p. 13.
2. Richard J. Kroening, Michael P. Volen, and David Bresler, "Acupuncture: Healing the Whole Person," in Herbert A. Otto and James W. Knight, eds. *Dimensions in Wholistic Healing: New Frontiers in the Treatment of the Whole Person.* Nelson-Hall: Chicago, 1979, p. 429.
3. Tara, "Oriental Medicine," p. 14.
4. William Tara, "Shiatsu," in Ann Hill, ed. *A Visual Encyclopedia of Unconventional Medicine.* Crown Publishers Inc.: New York, 1979, p. 65.
5. Sandy Newhouse and John Amodeo, "Native American Healing," in Edward Bauman, et al, eds. *The Holistic Health Handbook.* And/Or Press: Berkeley, California, 1978, p. 66.
6. Donald F. Sandner, "Navaho Indian Medicine and Medicine Men," in David S. Sobel, ed. *Ways of Health.* Harcourt Brace Jovanovich: New York, 1979, pp. 117, 121, 126-127.
7. Newhouse and Amodeo, p. 67.
8. C. H. Sharma, "Homeopathy," in Ann Hill, ed. *A Visual Encyclopedia of Unconventional Medicine.* Crown Publishers Inc.: New York, 1979, p. 22.
9. Sharma, p. 26.
10. David Anderson, Dale Buegel, and Dennis Chernin. *Homeopathic Remedies.* Himalayan International Institute: Honesdale, Pennsylvania, 1978, p. 3.
11. Richard Grossman. "Richard's Almanac," *Family Health,* April 1979, p. 57.
12. Harris L. Coulter, "Homeopathic Medicine," in David S. Sobel, ed. *Ways of Health.* Harcourt Brace Jovanovich: New York, 1979, p. 290.
13. Harris L. Coulter, "Homeopathy," in Leslie J. Kaslof, compiler and editor. *Wholistic Dimensions in Healing: A Resource Guide.* Doubleday and Company, Inc.: Garden City, New York, 1978, p. 48.
14. Anderson, et al, p. 3.
15. Linda Clark. *How to Improve Your Health: The Wholistic Approach.* Keats Publishing, Inc.: New Canaan, Connecticut, 1979, p. 82.

16. Nigel P. Castle, "Naturopathy," in Malcolm Hulke, ed. *The Encyclopedia of Alternative Medicine and Self-Help.* Schocken Books: New York, 1979, p. 138.

17. Ibid.

18. Mark Bricklin, ed. *The Practical Encyclopedia of Natural Healing.* Rodale Press, Inc.: Emmaus, Pennsylvania, 1976, p. 359; Castle, p. 139.

19. James A. Dyson and Carlotta Hollmann, "Anthroposophical Medicine," in Ann Hill, ed. *A Visual Encyclopedia of Unconventional Medicine.* Crown Publishers Inc.: New York, 1979, pp. 29-31.

20. John Addey, "Astrological Diagnosis," in Malcolm Hulke, ed. *The Encyclopedia of Alternative Medicine and Self-Help.* Schocken Books: New York, 1979, pp. 35-36; Mario Jones, "Astrology and Medicine," in Leslie J. Kaslof, compiler and editor. *Wholistic Dimensions in Healing: A Resource Guide.* Doubleday and Company, Inc.: Garden City, New York, 1978, pp. 162-164.

DIAGNOSTIC
METHODS

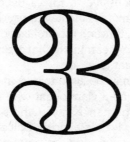

PSYCHIC DIAGNOSIS/HEALING

The word *psychic* is often used to refer to anything beyond the natural or known physical processes or to designate a person who demonstrates psychic powers and is sensitive to forces beyond the physical realm. Accordingly, the human mind is the key to psychic diagnosis/healing: in this method, one person, through total relaxation, total caring, and total love, is able to attune his or her mind to that of another human being and thereby diagnose and treat disease.[1]

The diagnosis may be ascertained in several ways. In some cases, the sensitive may be a clairvoyant who is able to literally "see" inside a patient, like a human X-ray. Others—called clair-audients—claim to hear voices that give a diagnosis. Still others, like Edgar Cayce, fall into a deep, trance-like sleep and answer questions about the patient's condition. Some people claim to have the ability to see, hear, and even communicate with those who are dead. At times, spirit guides have spoken through the psychic. One English sensitive enters a trance-like condition and goes on a "tour" of the patient's body with the aid of a spiritual guide.

There is no general agreement on the origin of psychic powers. Some advocates of psychic diagnosis/healing maintain that sensitives are born with the psychic gifts necessary for diagnosis and healing of patients, and that in some, this gift becomes stronger over the years.

24

Others appear to receive the gift later in life as the result of a traumatic experience, such as a severe illness or a particularly traumatic accident. Some claim that the ability can be developed in anyone—that it lies dormant in all of us. These individuals feel that any person who has great compassion for the ill possesses healing potential, but that the development of the gift is a matter of time, effort, and opportunity.

The way in which psychic healing/diagnosis is manifest varies from culture to culture, country to country, and belief system to belief system. Some rely on astronomy. In the Philippines, sensitives cover the patient with a sheet of white paper, coat it with oil, and watch for areas where the oil does not mark the paper; these areas indicate disease. In many belief systems, it is not even necessary for the patient to be present; the sensitive can make an accurate diagnosis by holding a picture of the patient, a personal letter from the patient, or some personal belonging of the patient's.[2] Still others can use telepathy to diagnose and heal. In this method, the psychic becomes the other person, feels the other's pains, and experiences the other's problems.

While studies and documentation of psychic healings and diagnoses are rare, one particularly amazing case involved a Brazilian healer named Arigó. An itinerant laborer who had completed only four years of primary school, Arigó was able to diagnose accurately using sophisticated medical terminology. A medical doctor who studied one thousand of Arigó's diagnostic statements expressed amazement at the sophistication and accuracy of the Brazilian healer's work.[3]

Others who use psychic diagnosis/healing believe that there is a psychic anatomy as well as a physical anatomy. This psychic anatomy is believed to exist in the form of energy emanations that surround living things, and it is often referred to as the *aura* (see the section on Kirlian photography in this chapter). Those with psychic powers are able to use the aura to determine the overall condition of the patient. A healthy aura, accordingly to those who practice psychic diagnosis/healing, surrounds the entire body and is about a foot in depth. In contrast, the aura of a sick person has gaps in places and may manifest the predominance of one particular color. One diagnostic method categorizes the colors and their meanings as follows:

BLACK: represents death, destruction, depreciation, or a state that precedes a constructive phase of life.
GRAY: represents boredom, malaise, fear, or anger.

BROWN: represents one who exercises or has enhanced physical abilities or one who has a state of low energy.

GREEN: represents one who is undergoing change in the areas of attitude, belief, or way of life.

BLUE: represents creativity, imagination, self-expression, repression, or the feminine.

YELLOW: represents intellect, a change from the unconscious to the conscious, refinement, or a growth of the mind.

ORANGE: represents healing or the masculine.

PINK: represents intuition or instinctive knowledge.

RED: represents emotions, warming to life, intensity, or passion.

PURPLE: represents spirituality or devotion.

GOLD: represents pure intuition, psychic prowess, self-knowledge, the masculine, cleansing or healing.

WHITE: represents the highest spiritual attainment, purification, or enlightenment.

These colors can be mixed, layered, blotchy, or chaotic in the diseased individual. Often an orange color is seen going from the healer to the person being healed. This signifies a feeling of warmth and attests that a healing is taking place by the transfer of energy from the healer to the healee.[4]

How does psychic diagnosis/healing work? According to some medical specialists, up to 80 percent of all human health problems can be classified as psychosomatic, either directly or indirectly.[5] If psychosomatic factors *are* a primary element in disease, then we have only our own minds to blame for our illnesses, and if we can effect a reversal of our own minds, then we can in essence obtain a cure, according to proponents of psychic healing. Many feel that the subconscious mind is one of man's greatest untapped natural resources. The basic question about psychic healing is whether healing is effected by the transfer of energy from the healer to the healee or whether it is caused by the powerful influence of the patient's own mind. One school of thought holds that psychic healing uses a combination of motivation, fear, commitment, and visual effects to achieve the profound physiological, metabolic, and psychological effects that can produce a remission or a cure.

Since most psychic healers are deeply religious, prayer also plays an important part in the diagnostic/healing process. Most believe that they are a channel for God's energy in the psychic process.[6]

Most psychic healers also have some physical contact with the patient. Such contact may consist of vigorous massage, manipulation of key pressure points in the body, or mere touching on the head. Those who practice surgery may use only an ordinary sharp-bladed knife (as did Arigó) or may part flesh with nothing more than their bare hands. An example of such bare-handed surgery was recorded on 8 millimeter film in the Philippines when Mrs. Ray Makela of Palo Alto, California, submitted to surgery to correct blocked nasal passages. Traditional surgeons in the United States had refused to perform the surgery because the prognosis was uncertain and the operation would leave her forehead hideously scarred.

Former *Time-Life* writer David St. Clair described the surgery as he saw it on film:

> In these pictures you can see Tony [Agpaoa, the psychic] smiling at the woman . . . his fingers suddenly part the flesh between her eyebrows. The blood runs down her face. His hands work quickly and he pulls out round bits of something that shines like fat globules . . . you note that he wears no gloves nor mask. He's peering into the wound, breathing in there, naked fingernails prodding. Then his hands come out and he swabs the already closed wound. There is no scar . . . her operation didn't take any longer to do than it took you to read about it.[7]

How is such healing possible? The author of the above passage claims that the intense energy emanating from the psychic's fingers resulted in a white light that heals.

Other purported examples of psychic healings have included psychic "injections" that pierced up to four layers of plastic hidden below the patient's clothing, even though no needle was used and the healer's hand was held two feet from the patient's body; sharp pain and a flow of blood when caused by a healer's hand held several feet from the patient's body; the dematerialization and rematerialization of cotton, and the insertion of the cotton into the patient's body without a body opening and with little apparent discomfort; and the extraction of teeth with no pain, by a healer who exerted only a slight pull with his bare hands.[8]

Healers are most abundant today in the United States, the Philippines, Brazil, and England, though they are of all races and colors and come from many religious affiliations. Both men and women are represented. Many have little formal education; indeed, some feel that a lack of education is an advantage to a psychic healer. The ability to heal may be developed at any time in the healer's life, and it does not necessarily decrease with age. The patient apparently does not have to have faith in the healer for a cure to take place, but most healers agree that it is helpful for the patient to have a strong personal belief system. Apparently the healing ability varies greatly between individual healers and is dependent on many factors, including desire for service, native abilities, experience, understanding of human nature, and attunement with the cosmos. Healers also have different specialties; for example, Tony Agpaoa was primarily involved in psychic surgery.[9]

IRIDOLOGY

The eyes have been called the *windows of the soul*. From this idea, Ignaz von Peczely formulated a technique which correlated the markings of the iris of the eye to diseases and conditions of specific organs of the body. He also analyzed the white portion of the eye, called the *sclera*, for an indication of the condition of some body organs.

From his early work and observations has come the modern, more refined practice of iridology.

> Iridology, or iris diagnosis, is the art and science practiced through the observation of the texture, pigmentation, and density of the iris whereby the physical condition and activity of all special organs and/or systems of the body are directly and most profoundly observed. Structural defects, chemical imbalances, toxemias (poisonous conditions), inherent weaknesses and predispositions, tensions, endocrine disorders, et al, are observed through direct iris examination.[10]

Thus, a miniature human body is correlated to parts of the iris, which can serve as a body map. Iridologists believe that the physical, mental, emotional, and spiritual aspects of man recorded in the eye lead to a unified understanding of the body.

Illness, injury, changes in body structures, and so on are also recorded by changes in the tissue of the iris. Such things as inflammations, build-up of drugs or other chemicals, abnormal acidity, and the progress of healing can be observed.[11] Iridology can also be used to

CHART TO IRIDOLOGY

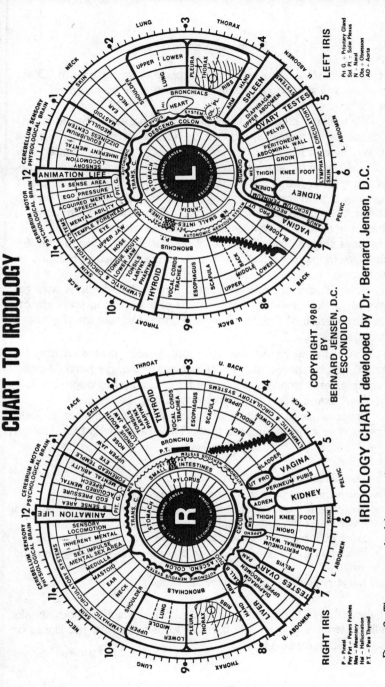

IRIDOLOGY CHART developed by Dr. Bernard Jensen, D.C.

COPYRIGHT 1980
BY
BERNARD JENSEN, D.C.
ESCONDIDO

P – Pineal
Pey Pat – Peyers Patches
Mes – Mesentery
Hal – Hallucination
P.T. – Para Thyroid

Pit G – Prituitary Gland
Sol. Pl – Solar Plexus
N – Naval
Obs – Obsession
AO – Aorta

Figure 2   The purpose of iridology is to determine the location of inflammation, the stage of inflammation, how it was caused, and the steps necessary to overcome it. The stages of inflammation in a specific area of the body are determined by the color changes in the corresponding specific area of the iris as shown in this chart.

predict disease, so it may serve as an early warning system. Often abnormalities will show up in the iris before actual physical symptoms of disease begin.

To make a diagnosis, iridologists compare the eye to charts which divide the iris radially and circularly. Radially, it is divided from one to sixty like the minutes in a clock face. Circularly, the iris is divided into three concentric rings with various subdivisions. "Each section corresponds to a specific part of the body, in much the same way as the foot is composed of a great many reflexology sections that also correspond to the various body parts and organs."[12] The diagrams in Figure 2 show how the iris is divided to represent the various parts of the body. Abnormalities such as cloudiness or discoloration, changes in density, and changes in pigment indicate problems or disease conditions in specific organs.

Sclera charts are also consulted. Lines, discolorations, scar tissue, and congested vessels in various parts of the sclera indicate abnormalities elsewhere in the body. Figures 3 and 4 indicate the diagnostic power of the sclera.

The iris may be observed through several means. It may be assessed simply by means of a 4x magnifying lens and a penlight or by more complex and technical equipment. For a very thorough, precise, and involved examination, a biomicroscope may be used.

Proponents of iridology conclude that iridology has definite advantages over other diagnostic tools. Their rationale is that through iridology:

- The whole body is visible at once on the iris.
- The technique for examination of the iris is noninvasive.
- The skills for iris examination and diagnosis are easily learned and transferred from patient to patient.
- Iridology provides an early warning system for disease detection.
- Iridology can act as an adjunct to other processes for diagnosis and healing.
- Large populations can be screened easily.[13]

They believe that iridology is a form of feedback in which the body speaks and tells us what is wrong. It is then up to us to resolve the illness or disease condition creatively.

KIRILIAN PHOTOGRAPHY

According to Lee R. Steiner, "Kirilian photography is a high-frequency, high-voltage photographic process in which part of the human body is imposed directly onto film, which, in turn, reproduces the electrical field changes that emanate from the human body (or any other living thing, including plants and animals)."[14]

The process was discovered by a Russian husband-and-wife team, Semyon and Valentina Kirilian, in the 1940s. In an experiment, they found that a spark jumped from an electrode on the equipment they were using to a patient lying close by. By placing a photographic plate between the electrode and the patient's hand, they observed that a luminescence followed the contours of the fingers, and that streams of energy emanated from the patient's fingertips. The process was later refined by the couple, and Semyon Kirilian described the results of the photography: ". . . galaxies of coloured lines, shining, twinkling; ghostly lights, bright multi-coloured flares, dim clouds, blazing violet, fiery flashes."[15] From observing these phenomena the Kirilians found that the size, structure, brightness, and colors differed from patient to patient.

At first it was thought that this remarkable occurrence came from changes in skin temperature, but this theory was disproved in time. The colorful phenomena were later termed an *aura* or a *corona,* and it was theorized to have been caused by an electromagnetic energy field occurring in a unified organism. Later it was postulated that there are characteristic aura for different states of health. Various mental states had a marked effect upon the quality and intensity of the emanation of energy. Many times a break in the aura itself indicated the presence of a physical abnormality. A disease condition of a specific organ showed as a lessening and darkening of the aural light over the area suffering the breakdown. Thus the Kirilians came to believe that the aura represents the "inner body" and is a reflection of the ills or well-being of the entire body and mind.

Though Kirilian photography is a relatively new procedure and is still in its infancy, it is purported to be useful for a variety of purposes:

1. It can be used to detect illness before physical symptoms appear.
2. It can evaluate the effectiveness of treatment by acupuncture, homeopathy, and other alternative healing methods.

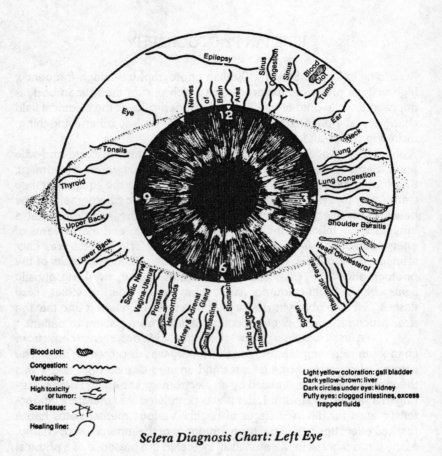

Labels on chart (clockwise from top): Epilepsy, Sinus Congestion, Sinus, Blood Clot, Tumor, Ear, Neck, Lung, Lung Congestion, Shoulder Bursitis, Heart Cholesterol, Rheumatic Fever, Spleen, Toxic Large Intestine, Stomach, Kidney & Adrenal Gland, Small Intestine, Hemorrhoids, Prostate, Vagina-Uterus, Sciatic Nerve, Lower Back, Upper Back, Thyroid, Tonsils, Eye, Nerves, of, Brain, Area

12, 9, 3, 6

Blood clot:
Congestion:
Varicosity:
High toxicity or tumor:
Scar tissue:
Healing line:

Light yellow coloration: gall bladder
Dark yellow-brown: liver
Dark circles under eye: kidney
Puffy eyes: clogged intestines, excess trapped fluids

Sclera Diagnosis Chart: Left Eye

Figures 3 and 4   Another way of checking for health problems is recommended by those who believe in sclerology. Overall body health is diagnosed by reading the lines and discolorations of the sclera, the white portion of the eye. (From *Bodymind*, by Ken Dychtwald, illustrated by Jad King. Illustration © 1977 by Jad King. Reprinted by permission of Pantheon Books, a Division of Random House, Inc., and Wildwood House Ltd.)

    3. It can be used for psychological detection of illness.
    4. It can alert others to residual toxic drug effects that may be present in the body.
    5. It can show the effects of parental conflict on children.
    6. It can show the psychological compatibility between people.[16]

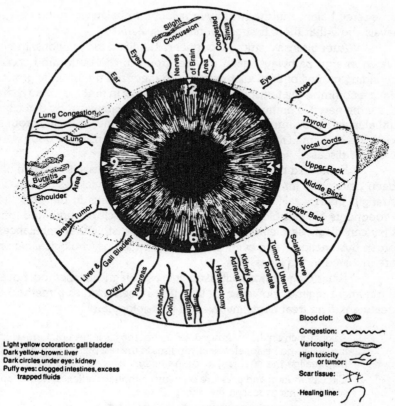

Light yellow coloration: gall bladder
Dark yellow-brown: liver
Dark circles under eye: kidney
Puffy eyes: clogged intestines, excess
        trapped fluids

Blood clot:
Congestion:
Varicosity:
High toxicity
  or tumor:
Scar tissue:
Healing line:

Sclera Diagnosis Chart: Right Eye

KINESIOLOGY

In 1965, Dr. George Goodheart, a respected United States chiropractor, discovered that relative muscle strength and tone—long used by chiropractors as indications of the range of motion over body joints—could also be used to diagnose disease in any organ of the body. Muscle-testing procedures are used to tap the innate intelligence of the body in order to assess the energy levels of life forces which control the body. Technically speaking, muscle strength and tone in the range of motion should reveal an energy balance in the healthy individual. Imbalances in the energy levels show that there is stress within the system.[17]

After intensive study, Goodheart identified the relationship between energy pathways, each muscle group in the body, and corresponding groups of particular organs. He theorized that muscle groups have a common relationship with internal organs in that they may share the same nervous pathways or the same energy pathways. By detecting imbalances and improper compensations in the muscle groups, Goodheart claimed to be able to diagnose which organs in the body were weak or diseased.

Expanded by many of Goodheart's colleagues, his research has been developed into the theory of kinesiology, a quick test of muscle strength that reveals instantaneously where problems in the body lie. Proponents of kinesiology claim that through muscle strength and tone they can diagnose dietary deficiencies, allergies, structural imbalances, organ dysfunctions, and even the extent to which psychological factors are involved in the illness.[18]

Kinesiology is normally used only as a diagnostic method, not as a treatment regime. However, of late, it has been used as a method of treatment. The treatments involved in kinesiology are:

1. A light touch on the neurovascular points, mostly in the cranium, which are switch-points for electrical impulses to the rest of the body. This can help realign the energy flow of the body.
2. Circular motion and pressure on neuro-lymphatic reflexes, nodes, and switch points to realign the energy flow.
3. Holding acupressure points.
4. Brushing meridian pathways lightly (for a definition of meridians, see the section on acupuncture Chapter 8).
5. Treating the origin and insertion of the muscle.
6. Dietary considerations.[19]

NOTES

1. Marika McCausland, "Psychic Diagnosis," in Ann Hill, ed. *A Visual Encyclopedia of Unconventional Medicine.* Crown Publishers Inc.: New York, 1979, p. 45.
2. McCausland, p. 45.

3. Francine Krisel. "Your Questions Answered on Psychic Healing," *Practical Psychology for Physicians,* June 1976, p. 74.
4. Amy Wallace and Bill Henken. *The Psychic Healing Book.* Dell Publishing Co., Inc.: New York, 1978, pp. 38-40.
5. Neil Chesanow. "Is it Time to Take Psychic Healing Seriously?" *Family Health,* January 1979, p. 24.
6. Krisel, p. 74.
7. Francine Krisel. "Your Questions Answered on Psychic Healing," *Practical Psychology for Physicians,* June 1976, pp. 74-75.
8. Meek, p. 42.
9. McCausland, p. 44.
10. Armand Ian Brint, "Iridology," in Edward Bauman, et al, eds. *The Holistic Health Handbook.* And/Or Press: Berkeley, California, 1978, p. 155.
11. Brint, p. 161.
12. Ken Dychtwald. *Bodymind.* Jove/HBJ: New York, 1977, pp. 230-231.
13. Brint, p. 162.
14. Lee R. Steiner. *Psychic Self-Healing for Psychological Problems.* Prentice-Hall, Inc.: Englewood Cliffs, New Jersey, 1977, p. 17.
15. John J. Williamson, "High Voltage Photography," in Malcolm Hulke, ed. *The Encyclopedia of Alternative Medicine and Self-Help.* Schocken Books: New York, 1979, p. 112.
16. Brian Snellgrove, "Kirlian Photography," in Ann Hill, ed. *A Visual Encyclopedia of Unconventional Medicine.* Crown Publishers Inc.: New York, 1979, pp. 48-49.
17. Brian H. Butler, "Applied Kinesiology," in Ann Hill, ed. *A Visual Encyclopedia of Unconventional Medicine.* Crown Publishers Inc.: New York, 1979, p. 44.
18. Brian H. Butler, "Applied Kinesiology," in Malcolm Hulke, ed. *An Encyclopedia of Alternative Medicine and Self-Help.* Schocken Brooks: New York, 1979, pp. 29-32.
19. Ibid.

THE
HUMAN HEALERS

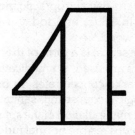

CHIROPRACTIC MEDICINE

Adapted from the Greek words meaning *manual medicine* or *manual practice,* chiropractic medicine was practiced by physicians as early as the time of Hippocrates. Modern-day chiropractic medicine was introduced by Daniel David Palmer in 1895, and today it is the largest drugless healing profession in the world.[1]

Chiropractic, in essence, is a form of therapy that is nonmedical and nonsurgical. No drugs are used, no medication is administered, no incision is made. Chiropractic concentrates on preventing and treating disease through psychological counseling, sanitation, hygiene, physical therapy, nutrition, and the manipulation of the spine and other joints.[2] It is believed that this regime helps restore normal function to the joints of the body and therefore helps the patient regain health.[3]

Chiropractic is much the same as osteopathic medicine; in fact, they evolved from the same practice, but there is a major difference between them: osteopaths believe that pain and disability result from pinched blood vessels, while chiropractors believe they are associated with pinched nerves caused by skeletal misalignment. Chiropractors center their work on the spine. Since the spine is the center of nervous transmission, they believe that manual adjustment can promote the health of tissues by promoting the health of the nerves.[4] Hence chiropractic deals mainly with diagnosis and correction of spinal and pelvic disorders such as misaligned vertebral discs, low back pain, and cervical, thoracic, and lumbar strains.

Like osteopaths, chiropractors rely on manual methods to treat patients, regardless of the proposed cause of the complaint. However, osteopaths use rhythmic movements and massage-like manipulation to restore circulation and health, while chiropractors use rapid thrusts and tugs to accomplish realignment.[5]

In examining a patient, the chiropractor concentrates on the spine, beginning with an X-ray. Proponents stress the importance of posture, symmetry, occupational factors, patient attitudes, weight, and evidence of underlying disease. The chiropractor also investigates injuries as the cause of joint abnormalities, abnormal muscle tone, and distortions that produce pain, nervous disturbances, circulatory congestion, malfunction of organs, and disease.[6]

Occasionally, a chiropractor may discover evidence of disease during an examination; in such cases, the patient is almost always referred to an orthodox physician for treatment.

Modern chiropractic medicine has evolved into a practice that involves a number of procedures that can be applied in many different ways, depending on the individual patient's condition. The most common method—and the one for which the chiropractor is best known—is a rapid manual thrust across a joint, designed to release a fixed (immobile) joint and restore full movement which will relieve tension on the surrounding nerve channels. Relief of this nervous irritation can return the joints and other affected organs to their original function, according to proponents.[7] Chiropractic practitioners are still developing techniques that employ more pressing and rolling and less emphasis on the better-known thrust technique.

Chiropractors perform other techniques not so well known to the public. Many give nutritional advice to patients; many others give advice about proper shoe fit and about changing usual working, sitting, and sleeping positions. Many chiropractors also use combinations of manipulation and vitamin therapy, ultraviolet and infrared light, whirlpool baths, hot and cold compresses, heel and sole lifts for shoes, acupuncture, and colonic irrigation.[8]

Advocates point out that chiropractors are trained in clinical and differential diagnosis, clinical neurology, and in the use of special instruments for diagnosis. The extent of the chiropractor's training does not enable him or her to practice obstetrics, psychiatry, surgery, or paramedical specialties; to reduce fractures or dislocations; to treat infectious or communicable diseases, cardiovascular diseases, pulmonary diseases, abdominal diseases requiring surgery, or tumors; prescribe, administer, or dispense drugs; use diagnostic tools involving chemicals or electrical devices; or use radiotherapy, fluoroscopy, or ionizing radiation. The chiropractor is allowed by law to use certain forms of X-ray as part of the examination process.[9]

CRANIAL TECHNIQUE

The cranium, or skull, is made up of eight bones joined together by hairline joints called *sutures.* Each suture has bony teeth that form a joint with the teeth of the adjacent suture. The teeth dovetail together much like those on a pair of gears.

These sutures are extremely close, but the constant movement and pressure exerted on them does cause them to move a little. Cranial technique proponents claim that in some cases, tiny pieces of the membrane covering the brain get caught and twisted in the sutures. When that happens, they say, the results can be devastating to health. They cite resulting disease conditions that range from toothache (not from decay but from grinding and twisting of the tooth on blood and nerve vessels) to migraine headaches and improper nerve functioning throughout the body.

According to proponents, approximately 95 percent of all people suffer from misalignment of the cranial bones and the resultant pressure and pinched membrane.[10]

The cranial technique calls on health practitioners to manipulate the cranial bones gently to relieve harmful pressure and produce slight movement of the sutures. While little movement results from the cranial technique, advocates claim that the movement is sufficient to produce relief from symptoms and related abnormalities caused by the misalignment.

DANCE THERAPY

For thousands of years dance has been viewed as a primal response to rhythm and music; magical properties have been attributed to it because at times dance seems able to put people in touch with themselves—a property that may help explain its healing qualities.

While the appreciation of dance dates back thousands of years, dance as a therapy had its beginnings in America shortly after World War II, when the climate of the mental health field began to change. American dancers and choreographers had long been known for creating dances based on personal struggles and emotional experiences, and the ideas for those dances came from the individual psyche. Following the war, increased funding and governmental encouragement spawned new and unconventional approaches to mental therapy, including dance as a group activity in the treatment of certain kinds of mental and emotional illness.

The notion received an added boost with the development of modern dance—an art form which came to prominence first in the 1940s and 1950s. Many of the modern dancers used their research into psychotherapy and their feelings about personal experiences to create their work, which evolved into a kind of therapeutic experience. The pioneers in modern dance—artists like Trudi Schoop, Liljan Espenak, Mary Whitehouse, and Blanche Evans—incorporated the theories of psychoanalysts like Freud, Adler, and Jung into their therapeutic dances.[11]

Official recognition of dance therapy as a healing technique came when administrators at St. Elizabeth Hospital in Washington, D. C., hired dancer Marian Chace to work with mental patients. Chace's reputation had been established by her studio work, but the results of her hospital work amazed the institution's officials. She was able to make contact with mutes and reach even the most stubborn and difficult of the mental patients by using dance to reflect patient conflicts and pain. Proponents of dance therapy say that she achieved success because she expanded the patients' self-awareness and created room for them to move and grow.

Advocates base their beliefs on the notion that there is an integral relationship between mind and body and that any movement that exercises and sculpts the body will have beneficial effect on the mind. Like music therapy, dance therapy is most often effective with those who are mentally, emotionally, and socially disturbed and those who have impaired communication abilities.

Proponents claim that dance provides a means of movement that is meaningful because it makes expression of self-knowledge and personal analysis easier. In other words, it reflects an awareness of the body and its sensations and emotions. Through dance movement, an individual can express hereditary heritage, experience, interpersonal behavior, and deep emotions.

One of the most valuable aspects of dance therapy, say advocates, is that it is an extremely effective way of acting out hidden hurts so the individual and the audience can get beneath the veneer of outward composure.[12] It is a valuable means of nonverbal communication.

The most widely accepted advantage of dance therapy, according to proponents, is that—like role playing—it helps an individual enter into an abnormal state so that hostilities, fears, and other symptoms can be acted out. Advocates point out that abnormal problems, previously undetected, can be revealed through a patient's dancing so a trained therapist can formulate a treatment.

Benefits of Dance

Proponents of dance therapy maintain that the benefits of dance are multifaceted.

Performed in a group (the usual mode of therapy), dance binds participants together into a functioning social unit, which, for some mental patients, is a novel experience. In addition, group dance therapy is done in a circle, which adds to the feeling of oneness and security. Dance therapy also teaches individuals to touch—both themselves and others—and thus extend themselves and make contact with others, again an extraordinary event for many mental patients, who have not learned or practiced this fundamental key to health.

Advocates of dance therapy maintain that it provides physical benefits that are in many ways as important as the emotional benefits. First, it provides the opportunity for exercise. Second, it involves muscle movement that helps relieve tension and releases vital energy. In essence, advocates claim that dance provides an ecstacy of movement which unifies the body and the spirit. Ultimately, dance provides for exercising the body's potentials and clearly defines its limitations—often significantly fewer than the patient previously believed. Dance therapy, say advocates, provides an accurate mental picture of the body that in turn forms the basis of the self-concept.

Proponents say that because the therapy sees the patient as an individual capable of unique movement, it has limitless possibilities as a therapeutic method. Advocates cite its possibilities as a diagnostic tool, a catharsis, an expression of fantasies, a form of regression, and a key to personality.[13]

ENCOUNTER

An outgrowth of the 1960s' questioning of the traditional values of society, encounter embodies many principles from other established therapies—including Gestalt, Zen, existentialism, and the theories of Freud, Lowen, and Reich. Basically, encounter therapy developed as a reaction against philosophies that attempted to make individuals conform to the status quo, or "to change themselves so they could accept the maladjustments of a sick society," in the words of encounter advocates. While many other forms of therapy advise people to adapt to society, encounter asks people to learn to accept themselves and come to terms with their own feelings.

A group therapy, encounter expects group members to express their feelings and accept responsibility for those feelings. Members are also required to relate honestly to other members of the group. Aside from these basic tenets, encounter groups have little structure: sessions progress as quickly and as far as creativity permits.

Usually, groups number about ten participants and a therapist, who establishes guidelines and helps direct discussions. In most cases the participants sit in a circle on the floor; the therapist guides them in introductory activities that promote acquaintance, helps group members express their feelings, and maintains control if some group members take sides against a single member.

Encounter sessions may be lengthy or brief—as short as one hour. Some are ongoing, and meetings are scheduled on a regular basis for months.

While encounter appears to uncover negative and painful feelings, advocates claim that its benefit lies in self-direction and growth that can facilitate mental and emotional healing and health.

MANIPULATIVE THERAPY

Manipulative therapy is sometimes considered a combination of osteopathic and chiropractic medicine because it relies on massage to promote health. Advocates say it may be the oldest form of medicine known to man.[14]

References to the Chinese system of massage are found in the writing of Kung Fu dating back to 3,000 B.C. Its practice in the Western world is attested to by writings in Greek; Hippocrates condemned hard and prolonged massage, but he instructed students that "moderate rubbing" causes tissues to grow.[15] He also maintained that massage could bind loose joints and loosen tight joints, an early reference to the benefits hailed by today's proponents of manipulative therapy.

References continue throughout history, from the time of the ancient Greeks to the nineteenth century, when massage was recognized as a remedial science in the United States after its 1877 introduction by Dr. S. W. Mitchell. The first professional organization practicing manipulative therapy was formed by a group of British women in 1894; by 1920 several other organizations had been formed, several books had been published, and schools were to be found in most major cities throughout England. Many of these schools still exist and train advocates in the principles of manipulative therapy.

While the practitioner embraces some of the techniques of chiropractic and osteopathic medicine, advocates of manipulative therapy do not believe the problem lies in either pinched blood vessels or pinched nerves. Some of their efforts center on the joints, but much of the therapy concerns itself with the soft tissues.

Four main techniques are used:

• *Effleurage.* A process of stroking the skin lightly with the palms, effleurage is commonly applied on the back to improve circulation and induce relaxation. The practitioner exerts slight pressure while moving in wide stroking motions, searching for lesions or tenderness.

• *Petrissage.* This manipulation of the soft tissues of the shoulders, neck, and upper back improves circulation, hence nourishment, of both blood and lymph tissues. The practitioner of petrissage ("picking up") uses a combination of techniques—usually rolling, wringing, and gentle kneading.

• *Friction.* The practitioner usually uses a thumb to create deep friction around joints and along the spine, where it is especially helpful, say advocates, in toning the muscles and ligaments so important to support of the spinal column.

• *Traction.* To ease tension on the neck, the practitioner maintains gentle manual traction, often in combination with friction therapy on the scalp at the base of the skull. Muscles supporting the neck and head are worked with petrissage and friction to complete the treatment.

MASSAGE/SOMATOTHERAPY

Like manipulative therapy, massage therapy (often referred to as *somatotherapy*) is derived from massage, which, proponents believe, is the oldest form of medicine known to man. Begun in the Orient, the therapy quickly spread to the West and is currently practiced throughout the world.

While the principles of massage are the same, the practice varies slightly. Oriental massage, often called *amma massage,* emphasizes the meridians through which the vital energy force of the body is channeled, the same principles that form the basis of acupuncture. Western concepts of massage, on the other hand, emphasize upward motions toward the patient's heart.

The purposes of massage differ, too, according to geographical location. Oriental massage is geared toward giving relief from fatigue, sluggishness, stiff shoulders, headaches, chilliness in the hands and feet, and swelling. Conversely, Western massage concentrates on the nerves, joints, muscles, and endocrine system and treats disorders like geriatric stiffness, stroke, poliomyletis, numbness and pain in the arms, pain in the stomach and intestinal tract, and chronic constipation.[16]

The underlying principle of massage is that all information received by the mind must be received by the body first, and the way the body acts will affect the information the mind ultimately receives. The body affects the mind, and the mind affects the body. Massage attempts to unify, coordinate, and integrate body and mind by the stimulating or inhibiting nerves or muscles on the theory that every part of the body is controlled by a spinal nerve. Gentle pressure of the fingertips is used to suppress nerve function, and heavier pressure is used to stimulate. By relieving nerve transmission, pain, numbness, chilling, and stiffness in the skin and muscles are mitigated, and the internal organs are returned to a sound and healthy condition. In summary, then, massage can stimulate the spinal and other nerves, inhibit the spinal and other nerves, release muscle contractions, and neutralize or regulate blood supply. These all help to increase the body's resistance to disease and to control disease or debilitating conditions that may already be present.

Ten basic techniques make up the principles behind massage therapy:

1. *Light pressure.* Light pressure improves the circulation of blood and lymph, provides stimulation for nerves, muscles, and internal organs, and promotes healthy skin.
2. *Rubbing and kneading.* Used mostly on muscle tissue, rubbing and kneading requires the practitioner to hold the muscle and use the palms and balls of the fingers to perform circular movements.
3. *Pressing.* Pressing is accomplished by pressing the tissues with the palms, thumbs, and fingers.
4. *Vibration.* A form of massage called *vibration* is accomplished by holding the muscle and shaking it lightly. Vibration stimulates blood flow and nerve force.
5. *Tapping.* Tapping a muscle with both hands breaks up muscle congestion, relieves muscle spasms, relaxes strained muscles, and builds red blood cells.
6. *Circular pressure.* Applying pressure in decreasing concentric circles relaxes the tissues following the previous techniques.
7. *Effleurage.* Effleurage consists of long, continuous stroking of the limbs, back, and torso. By placing both hands palm down, one on top of the other, the practitioner can promote lymphatic drainage, muscular relaxation, and circulation.
8. *Friction.* A technique that opens the pores, brings blood to the skin surface, and produces tone and color of the skin, friction is accomplished by brisk sliding or rubbing movements of the hands. Some practitioners use oil to reduce abrasion or irritation to the skin.
9. *Touching.* The practitioner holds his hands in one position on the patient's body, to effect an exchange of energy.

10. *Twisting.* Wringing sections of the skin stimulates nerve reaction and brings blood to a localized area of the skin.

MUSIC THERAPY

Proponents of music therapy maintain that music has a powerful effect on the body and the mind, and that it can be used as an effective form of therapy.[17] Music has the ability to penetrate different levels of consciousness, say proponents, and it is an expressive art that speaks to the physical, mental, and emotional aspects of every human being, encompassing the full range of human experience and serving many purposes in man's existence.

Seven basic qualities of music make it particularly well-suited for therapy:[18]

- It is a form of nonverbal communication between individuals or in a group.
- Music is flexible and can be used in many ways by many different people. Anyone from an infant to a centenarian can enjoy music. Anyone from the most brilliant pianist to a retarded child can produce it.
- Music is a socializing agent that brings people together.
- Music evokes tender emotions and encourages the expression of those emotions.
- Music itself is enjoyable—it provides an instant gratification of desires and needs.
- Music can produce an emotional purging, or catharsis, in many individuals.
- Music has a sedative effect that can, in many cases, ease pain and grief.

Five elements are contained in sound and music: pitch, duration, tone, color, and volume. Each affects the whole person—mind, body, and emotions—in an individual way, so responses to music depend entirely on the person who listens to or produces the music. But the specific, standard effect of music that is valuable in therapy is its ability to integrate and unify the spheres of mind, body, and emotion within man.

Music therapy is currently being used to open communication for those who cannot communicate, those who are mentally and emotionally disturbed and who can communicate only on a limited basis because it tends to restore and develop the perceptual, physical, and mental contacts necessary for communication.

Advocates claim that music therapy has also enjoyed some success in helping rehabilitate people socially, because it can help people feel useful and needed and can help people learn to relate to a group when it is used properly. Music has been used with some success to help women overcome the fear of the childbirth experience, and it has been used on a limited basis with asthma patients in an attempt to arrest the progression of the disease with the sedative qualities of music.

Music therapy can be either active, as when the patient uses an instrument or his own voice to produce music or receptive, as when the patient listens to music produced by others. Proponents say that active music therapy is particularly useful in helping patients learn to express themselves, while receptive therapy has been successful in changing patients' moods and behavior.[19]

OSTEOPATHY

While different forms of manipulative therapy were used in many parts of the world from the time of Hippocrates, the first formal description of an entire system of healing by manipulation was given in 1876 by Dr. Andrew Taylor Still, a Missouri physician who had helplessly watched three of his sons die from meningitis. Still spent sixteen years of study and experiment before he came up with his theories, and it was almost twenty years later, in 1897, that the first college of osteopathy was established in Kirksville, Missouri.[20] By the time Still died at the age of eighty-nine, osteopathy was recognized in every state and had been awarded equal recognition with orthodox medicine.

"Bone setting" is similar to chiropractic, where bones are realigned. While bone setting was a common practice among the physicians of Still's day, it was mostly used to realign broken bones and to break down lesions that occur around joints and old fracture sites. Osteopathy was more. Advancing the theory that bodily structure and function are completely interdependent, Still maintained that if the structure of the body is altered in any way, the function immediately alters as well. Conversely, any alteration in function will cause an immediate alteration in structure.

Osteopathic physicians believe that alterations are caused by the biped stance of human beings plus traumas that occur in everyday living. The combination of these factors causes mechanical disturbances and imbalances, especially in the pelvic, spinal, and cranial areas. These imbalances create abnormal reflex patterns and arterial compression that cause interference with blood flow and normal nerve transmission. Osteopaths maintain that when blood flow is normal, structure and function are likely to be normal[21] and that it is impossible to restore full health—physical and mental—without correcting anatomical derangements. Although the spine and its abnormal shifts are osteopaths' major concern, they are also concerned with the structure and function of the ribs, pelvis, and thorax, as well as soft tissue like muscles and ligaments.

After taking a thorough case history from the patient, the osteopath proceeds with a physical examination that is peculiar to osteopathy. Instead of restricting himself to the area of obvious disease or pain, the osteopath proceeds to examine the patient's entire system. The patient lies on a couch while the osteopath moves each joint through its range of motion. The arms and legs are used as levers for probing and manipulating to restore full motion to each joint. If a joint is stiff or frozen, the osteopath "opens" it by manipulation while exerting pressure on the spine. At this point osteopathy differs greatly from chiropractic medicine, as the chiropractor relies on a direct thrust to the vertebrae while the patient is lying prone and still.

Osteopathy is not restricted to treatment of spinal misalignments or lesions. It has been successful in the treatment of a wide range of physical complaints. Osteopaths also treat infectious disease by manipulation, which is used to get the lymph moving through the lymph nodes so more antibodies are manufactured and mobilized to fight the infection.[22]

If the disease problem (whether infectious or not) is of recent origin, only one or two visits are usually needed for correction. If the problem is a longstanding one, the body has often adapted to the misalignment and will generally slip back out of alignment within a short period of time, necessitating a number of osteopathic treatments over a period of weeks or months. In chronic cases that have developed over a number of years, osteopaths frequently recommend surgery or other forms of orthodox treatment.[23] In addition, osteopaths uphold the basic hygiene and health practices which contribute to health, disease, and disease treatment.

REFLEXOLOGY

Many acupuncture and shiatsu principles are involved in reflexology which employs massage of certain points on the feet which advocates believe correspond to particular body functions and organs. Like practitioners of shiatsu and acupuncture, practitioners of reflexology believe that energy flows through the body along meridians that have their terminal points in the feet. A healthy flow and balance of energy through these meridians is responsible for the health of the individual, according to proponents of the theory.

Practitioners believe that reflex points on the top and bottom of the feet correspond to 72,000 nerve endings that in turn are connected to body parts and organs in the trunk and head. (See Figures 5, 6, 7, and 8. They are all taken from "Reflexology," in Edward Bauman, et al., *The Holistic Health Handbook.* Copyright © 1978 by Marlyn Amann. Reprinted by permission from *The Holistic Health Handbook,* And/Or Press, Inc.) Also called *zone therapy,* reflexology was practiced by the ancient Chinese, by tribes in Kenya, and by some tribes of American Indians.[24]

Proponents claim that properly performed reflexology can also serve as a diagnostic tool. If an organ is healthy and functions properly, the corresponding reflex point on the foot is similarly good. Conversely, if an organ does not function optimally, the foot zone will become sensitive to touch. Reflex areas that are tender to the touch signal disease or deterioration of the corresponding organ or function. When an organ or part of the body is malfunctioning or unhealthy, the corresponding point on the foot is said to feel as if there is a needle or broken glass stuck in it or as if there are grains of sand under the foot. Some reflexologists feel that this sandy sensation is caused by uric acid or calcium crystals accumulating at the reflex area site. The concentration of these crystals indicates to them that certain organs are not able to carry on complete metabolic processes. They believe that the uric acid and calcium signal the accumulation of waste products and indicate malfunction.[25] It is thought that the amount of discomfort varies according to the severity of the condition.

Once areas of tenderness—hence disease—have been identified, reflexologists claim to be able to release tension and encourage full blood circulation using only the hands (primarily the thumbs and fingers) to massage various points on the feet and stimulate full blood circulation

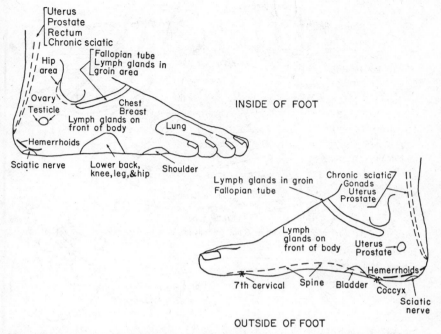

Figure 5 Advocates of foot reflexology believe that specific areas on the tops and bottoms of the feet correspond to various organs and systems through thousands of nerve endings that make the connecting links.

to the organs which are linked to the reflex areas of the feet. Massage and the application of constant pressure and rotation are said to stimulate not only the circulation but also the nerve endings that activate sluggish glands and organs to increase their function and remedy the condition.[26]

Whether the foot is rubbed, stroked, kneaded, or massaged, the constant pressure is necessary. It may vary in intensity to produce different reactions and different remedial effects. Generally, firm pressure is best for therapy, but it should not be so firm that pain or discomfort is created.

Lew Connor and Linda McKim describe an all-purpose reflexology massage that can be used for prevention of disease and general health maintenance: It begins with a light rubbing, stroking, kneading, or massage of the foot and moves to the solar plexus reflex, which helps to release tension and promote a general feeling of well-being. The toes,

51

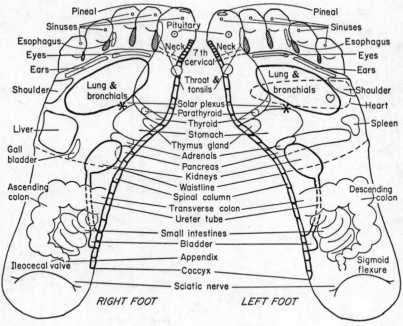

Pineal — Pituitary — Pineal
Sinuses — Neck — 7th cervical — Neck — Sinuses
Esophagus — Esophagus
Eyes — Eyes
Ears — Ears
Throat & tonsils
Shoulder — Lung & bronchials — Lung & bronchials — Shoulder
Heart
Solar plexus
Parathyroid
Liver — Thyroid — Spleen
Stomach
Gall bladder — Thymus gland
Adrenals
Pancreas
Kidneys
Ascending colon — Waistline — Descending colon
Spinal column
Transverse colon
Ureter tube
Small intestines
Bladder
Ileocecal valve — Appendix — Sigmoid flexure
Coccyx
Sciatic nerve

RIGHT FOOT   LEFT FOOT

Figure 6

which represent the head and its accompanying organs, are next, and the practitioner proceeds down the foot, working from the outside to the inside. The colon area, located approximately in the middle of the foot, should be manipulated from the center inside to outside and down toward the heel. The heel is the last to be massaged, and it should be worked on the bottom from the outside toward the center.

The top of the foot is massaged from the outside of the heel to the inside and between the toes. The massage is finished by gently stroking the tops of the feet.[27]

Proponents of reflexology claim that people of all ages benefit from the massage, and the age and condition of the patient determine the extent and amount of pressure exerted. Most who experience foot reflexology, say advocates, find that it relaxes tension, increases circulation, and promotes an overall feeling of good health. Reflexologists point out that in situations where the feet cannot be massaged, many of the same results can be obtained by massaging the hands in the same manner.

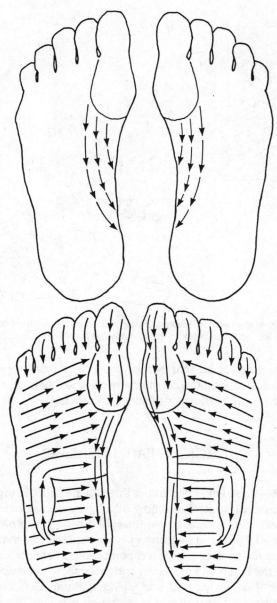

Figure 7 Some advocates of foot reflexology suggest foot manipulations to prevent
disease and maintain health. One approach is to massage the bottom of the foot as
illustrated above—by starting with the toes and moving down the foot—ending with the
heel—always working from the outside of the feet and working toward center.

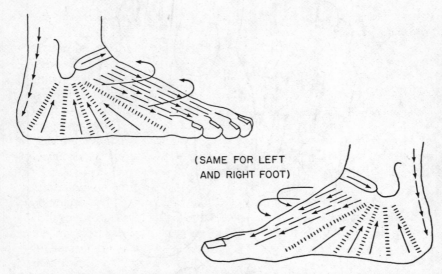

(SAME FOR LEFT
AND RIGHT FOOT)

Figure 8   The next approach is to massage the top of the foot, moving from the heel area to the front of the foot and then between the toes. Always move in the directions indicated.

Advocates claim that reflexology brings relief for congestion (especially sinus congestion), migraine headaches, pancreas problems, liver disorders, constipation, and kidney disorders.[28]

RELIGIOUS/FAITH HEALING

Faith healers—those who effect a cure through the faith of the patient and the practitioner without medication or surgery—have recently come under scientific investigation by members of the medical profession.[29] As a result, some scientists say emerging evidence indicates that actions of the mind and the spirit can have a dramatic impact on physical health.

"In the beginning physician and priest were indivisible, all healing divine."[30] People felt that underlying spiritual disorders were the cause of illness, and thus, the role of the church was "to preach the kingdom of God, and to heal the sick."[31] Hence, "the religious task and the healing task are essentially the same: to release the individual from the

54

destructive realities and bring him or her into a relationship with the protective, positive, and healing realities."[32]

The mind's powers have been used for centuries to overcome physical disease (as the miraculous healings at the shrine at Lourdes, France attest), and faith healers attempt to channel those healing mental powers. The fundamental difference between religious and psychic healing is that religious and faith healers claim that their power comes from God or other divine sources and that the healer and the recipient of the healing are instruments of divine power. In religious healing, there may be no need of a healer or an intermediary. The divine power may effect the healing directly.

Many people believe that emotions such as resentment, hatred, jealousy, and other such negative feelings can be traced to the beginning of life. These negative feelings create psychological scars which result in physical and emotional illness. To rid the individual of these scars and the resulting illness, advocates suggest that Jesus Christ becomes the catalyst who is all-forgiving and loving. Inner healing results if men open their hearts and minds to Christ, accept His love and forgiveness, and in turn love and forgive others who have hurt them.[33]

Central to faith healing is meditation and prayer, which is aimed at helping the patient relax. Physiologically, scientists have learned that such meditation slows the heartbeat, eases muscle tension, and lowers blood pressure, resulting in therapy for a variety of stress-related diseases. Three University of California physicians demonstrated that hopeful thoughts may even cause the brain to secrete its own powerful pain-killing drugs, drugs closely related to morphine, which are called endorphins.[34]

While various methods may be employed by faith healers, one of the most common is laying on of hands: the healer's hands are placed, palm down, on top of the patient's head, shoulders, or waist. The concept of the laying on of hands is based on the belief that the human body has a vital energy force flowing through it and that every healthy person has an excess of energy—more than he needs for his own purposes. The healer tries to direct and transmit this excess energy, or healing force, into the body of the ill person, who has less than optimal energy, due to the illness. Advocates suggest that this healing force corresponds to that healing force used by Jesus Christ.

To find the part of the body to which the energy should be

transferred, the healer puts himself in a state of meditative consciousness sometimes referred to as "healing meditation." The healer then "listens" as his hands scan the patient's body from a distance. When the hands encounter areas of accumulated tension or blocked energy flow, the healer lays his hands on the patient's body and tries to redirect his energies to these parts. As he does so, his mind and faith are focused on the healing taking place.[35]

Although most healers utilize this laying on of hands and heal through the fingers or palms, some do not touch the patient. Many patients report that physical sensations occur during the healing, whether they were touched or not. Some of the sensations have been described as cold, hot, prickly, painful, and creaking (like creaking joints). Generally, the healer keeps his hands in position over the abnormal part of the body until the patient indicates that these sensations have disappeared.[36]

Laying on of hands is engaged in by clergy in several leading churches and was also practiced by Ruth Carter Stapleton, sister of former President Jimmy Carter.

ROLFING

Sometimes referred to as "structural processing," rolfing was developed in the United States in the late 1930s by Ida Rolf as a form of deep massage to realign the body to its proper posture.[37] The aim of rolfing today is the achievement of a structurally balanced body: knees vertical over the ankles, hip joints vertical over the knees, shoulders vertical over the hip joints, and ears vertical above the shoulders.[38]

Central to the theory of rolfing is the relationship of the individual with the gravity that rules the universe: when the posture is out of alignment, say advocates, the individual is bent over by gravity; when the posture is properly aligned, the individual is supported by gravity, and all systems are freer to function properly. An unbalanced body is unstable and causes energy loss so that tremendous muscular strength must be expended to keep it from toppling. Proponents say it takes less energy to move a body that is aligned along a vertical axis.[39]

How does misalignment occur in the first place? Proponents of rolfing believe that the mind and body are interconnected, and that past traumatic experiences reveal themselves in the posture. Further, these repressed experiences from the past cause unconscious muscle tension that causes the body to move out of a state of natural alignment and vitality into a state of overall inflexibility and gravitational imbalance.[40] In addition to limited range of movement and inflexibility, the traumatic experiences and the accompanying muscle tension, cause restriction of circulation, inefficient organ function, and muscle overuse or underuse. Other factors can add to postural misalignment: general patterns of walking, sitting, and sleeping can cause permanent postural distortions. Accidents like falls and athletic injuries can also impair posture and cause alignment difficulties.

Rolfing is a process of organizing and balancing the body left to right, front to back, top to bottom, and inside and out along a vertical line so one is supported by gravity instead of hampered by it. Unlike osteopathy and chiropractic medicine, which concentrate on the realignment of bones and joints, rolfing concentrates on the alteration of soft organs, muscles, ligaments, and fascia (the envelope of connective tissue that houses the structures of the body). Strong manipulation is exerted to move and stretch these tissues. The massage starts with the surface of the body and goes on to the deeper structure. Fingers, knuckles, and elbows are used, and the massage can be painful. Generally ten treatment sessions are required over a period of five to ten weeks.[41]

In addition to physical benefits, there are many psychological benefits derived from rolfing. It has been said by proponents that the deep massage helps rid the subconscious of the traumatic experiences from the past that have contributed to the posture misalignment. They claim that during the sessions individuals relive the experiences and that this dispels the feelings of anxiety and frees the body of their effects. This permits the consciousness to be expanded.[42]

It has been said that the rolfing process is accompanied by a great emotional and energetic release and purge that may take the form of expressions of deep sadness, fear, joy, and other unresolved emotions. For example, when the back is rolfed, the individual is likely to experience the vestiges of past rage and anger. Rolfing the jaws releases the emotion of sadness. When the hips are rolfed, past emotions connected with sexuality are released. The shoulders are often sources of past burdens and stressful responsibilities, so when deep massage is applied to them, release of emotions connected with burdens and stressful responsibilities are released.[43]

Once this emotional and energetic release takes place, the

body's vital energy flow is again established, and an integration of the body and mind is achieved.

SHIATSU
(PRESSURE THERAPY)

A predominant form of Oriental medicine, shiatsu, *finger pressure,* uses firm pressure to various points on the skin known as pressure points. The origin of this practice is the instinctive human response to pain: to touch the place that hurts. Shiatsu amplifies this principle by using the hands in areas where vital energy, or *ki*, is strongest.

Ki follows along meridian paths, and the pressure points along the meridians are the same points used in acupuncture (hence the references to shiatsu as *acupressure massage*).[44] When these pressure points are stimulated by thumbs or fingers, body function and physiology, particularly organ function, are affected. The goal of shiatsu is to promote better health by stimulating the flow of ki energy in the body.

Families in the Orient have used shiatsu on each other for centuries, but it was not introduced in the West until the latter half of this century. Thousands have learned it and now practice it in the home. Shiatsu can be done anywhere, alone or with another person. It does not require hours of strain or effort to accomplish its results. Amateurs who practice on members of their own family for simple relief from pain or fatigue have experienced substantial success. Advanced practitioners claim to be able to treat specific illnesses and stimulate specific organs through massage of specific pressure points.

According to practitioners, the individual giving the shiatsu massage should be calm, responsive, and in good health; and should act on personal intuition. The individual receiving the massage should wear loose-fitting, lightweight clothing of natural fibers if clothing is worn at all. If the person receiving the massage is seated, the spine should be completely straight. The room should be free of distractions, quiet, and simply furnished. Pressure should be geared to each individual, but heavy pressure should never be exerted on the abdomen, face, or behind the joints of the knees or elbows. Application of pressure on a particular point should be maintained for five to seven seconds three or four times during the massage session. The pressure and massage should be given by using the thumbs; index, middle, and ring fingers; and the palm of the hand.[45]

According to practitioners, pain felt along any of the meridians during shiatsu massage indicates stagnation of ki to the corresponding organ. After several sessions of shiatsu, the ki should flow freely, and the pain should disappear. The most common meridians and their corresponding organs include the upper outside surface of the arm and the area between the thumb and index finger in the fleshy part of the hand (the large intestine), under the fleshy part of the calf between the knee and ankle (the liver), along the outside of the leg from the pelvis to the knee (gall-bladder), under the shin bone on the inside of the leg between the ankle and the knee (the spleen), just to the outside of the front ridge of the shin bone from the knee to the ankle (the stomach), the top inside surface of the calf on top of the muscle (the kidneys), the bottom outside surface of the arm and the shoulder blades (the heart), the upper inside surface of the arm and the area beneath the clavicle on the upper chest (the lungs), the bottom inside surface of the arm from the little finger to the armpit (the small intestine), and the middle of the back of the thigh and both sides of the coccyx (the urinary bladder).[46]

Advocates claim that shiatsu is effective in correcting faulty circulation, reducing muscle pain, and reducing the amount of lactic acid to the muscles, which can, in turn, help decrease fatigue, tension, and soreness in the muscles. Shiatsu has also been effective in treating high blood pressure, arthritis, diabetes, rheumatism, stomach and intestinal problems, migraine headache, neuralgia, insomnia, and problems with overweight, according to proponents.[47]

Advocates stress that shiatsu should be practiced in connection with proper diet, activity, and attitude; good health habits should be consistently practiced for the shiatsu to be effective. Most practitioners strive to use shiatsu as a preventive, rather than healing, method.

TEMPOROMANDIBULAR JOINT TECHNIQUE

First formulated and used with denture wearers, the temporomandibular joint technique (TMJ) is based on the theory that much stress results from misalignment of the temporomandibular joint, the joint which joins the jawbone and skull.

Dentists who formulated the TMJ technique feel that as much as 50 percent of the body's stress load can be decreased by maintaining the proper position of the jaw.[48] Stress caused by misalignment of the jaw can be heightened during the chewing process, and unless the jaw is in a proper position, the stress is not even relieved during sleep, according to advocates. The result? The body is subject to constant stress.

Advocates of the TMJ technique feel that misalignment of the jaw can affect almost every aspect of life. Particular conditions that relate to jaw misalignment include pain in the neck, head, ears, and jaw; ringing in the ears; deafness; joint tenderness; dizziness; dental malocclusion (crooked teeth); some neuromuscular conditions; and osteoarthritis.[49]

When practitioners manipulate the jaw, the joints are brought back into alignment. With proper alignment, say proponents, the jaw muscles are relieved of their need to compensate, and they coordinate better with other muscles in the head and neck, thus relieving tension.

NOTES

1. Alan C. Breen, "Chiropractic," p. 73 in Ann Hill, editor, A Visual Encyclopedia of Unconventional Medicine (New York, New York: Crown Publishers, Inc., 1979).

2. Brent Q. Hafen, Alton L. Thygerson, and Ronald L. Rhodes, Prescriptions for Health (Provo, Utah: Brigham Young University Press, 1977), p. 240.

3. R. Gerald Cooper, "Chiropractic," p. 59 in Malcolm Hulke, editor, The Encyclopedia of Alternative Medicine and Self-Help (New York: Schocken Books, 1979).

4. Breen, p. 73.

5. Ibid., p. 74.

6. Cooper, p. 59.

7. Breen, p. 74.

8. Joseph B. Treaster, "Chiropractic Comes of Age," Family Health, December 1978, p. 28.

9. Hafen et. al, pp. 240-241.

10. Major B. DeJarnette, "Cranial Technique," p. 84 in Leslie J. Kaslof, compiler and editor, Wholistic Dimensions in Healing: A Resource Guide (Garden City, New York: Doubleday and Company, Inc., 1978), p. 133.

11. Claire Schmais, "Dance Therapy: The Psychotherapeutic Use of Movement," pp. 229-231 in Kaslof.

12. Esther C. Frankel, "Dance Therapy," p. 121 in Mark Bricklin, editor, The Practical Encyclopedia of Natural Healing (Emmaus, Pennsylvania: Rodale Press, Inc., 1976).

13. Felicity Ling, "Dance Therapy," p. 228 in Hill.
14. K. Woodward, "Manipulative Therapy," pp. 82-83 in Hill.
15. Ibid.
16. Katsusuki Serizawa, "Massage," p. 207 in Kaslof.
17. Juliette Alvin, "Music Therapy," p. 134 in Hulke.
18. Ibid.
19. Alvin, p. 135.
20. Stephen Pirie, "Osteopathy," p. 69 in Hill.
21. Ibid.
22. James W. McCullagh, "Chiropractic," p. 73 in Hill.
23. Pirie, pp. 71-72.
24. Doreen E. Bayly, "Reflexology," p. 61 in Hill.
25. Lew Connor and Linda McKim, "Reflexology," p. 183 in Edward Bauman, Armand Ian Brint, Lorin Piper, and Pamela Amelia Wright, *The Holistic Health Handbook* (Berkeley, California: The AND/OR Press, 1978).
26. Ibid.
27. Ibid., pp. 184-185.
28. Martine Faure-Alderson, "Reflexology," p. 172 in Hulke.
29. "Science Takes a New Look at Faith Healing," *U.S. News and World Report,* February 12, 1979, p. 68.
30. "Religion and Medicine Draw Closer," *Medical World News,* December 25, 1978, p. 26.
31. Luke 9:2.
32. Morton T. Kelsey, "Faith: Its Function in the Wholistic Healing Process," p. 219 in Herbert A. Otto and James W. Knight, editors, *Dimensions in Wholistic Healing: New Frontiers in the Treatment of the Whole Person* (Chicago, Illinois: Nelson-Hall, 1979).
33. E. M. Oakley, "Focusing on Health, Not Illness," *New Realities,* April 1979, p. 24.
34. *U. S. News,* p. 69.
35. *U. S. News,* p. 69; Dolores Krieger, Erik Peper, and Sonia Ancoli, "Therapeutic Touch: Searching for Evidence of Physiological Change," *American Journal of Nursing,* April 1979, p. 660.
36. Elizabeth Baerlein, "Hand Healing," p. 89 in Hulke.
37. "Rolfing," p. 80 in Hill.
38. Richard Grossman, "Richard's Almanac," *Family Health,* April 1979, p. 53.
39. "Rolfing," pp. 80-81.
40. Ken Dychtwald, *Bodymind* (New York: Jove/Harcourt Brace Jovanovich, 1977), p. 12.
41. "Rolfing," pp. 80-81.

42. Nathaniel Lande, "A Comprehensive Overview of Today's Life-Changing Philosophies," *Mindstyles/Lifestyles,* p. 177.
43. Dychtwald, p. 14.
44. William Tara, "Oriental Medicine," p. 65 in Hill.
45. William Tara, "Shiatsu," p. 64 in Hill.
46. Ibid.
47. John Newton, "Shiatsu Massage," p. 177 in Hulke.
48. Willie B. May, "The Position of the Mandible (Lower Jaw) as It Relates to Stress in the Human System," p. 86 in Kaslof.
49. Harold T. Perry, "Temporomandibular Joint Technique," p. 88 in Kaslof.

PHYSICAL
REGIMENS

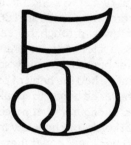

THE ALEXANDER TECHNIQUE

The Alexander Technique, sometimes mistakenly assumed to be simple posture exercises, began as one man's effort to improve his own health. F. Matthias Alexander, born in Australia in 1869, began experiencing severe voice problems midway through his career as an actor. After countless trips to countless doctors who were unable to help him, Alexander set out to find out for himself why his voice was malfunctioning.

He discovered that he had the habit of pulling his head back and sucking in his breath whenever he began to speak—and the combination depressed his vocal cords. He figured that he could not directly control the depression of his vocal cords, but he knew that he could change the way he held his head and neck and could thereby improve the muscle tone in his chest and improve his breathing.

His discoveries and his techniques—which centered on using the self—were successful, and he began teaching his technique to others in 1894.

At first, his technique went without recognition or support from members of the medical profession. In 1904 he moved to London, where he finally published *Man's Supreme Inheritance*—a book that attracted attention and caused him to steadily grow in popularity. After the outbreak of World War I, he began spending half his time in the United States. His second book, *Constructive Conscious Control of the Indi-*

vidual (1924), attracted further attention. Finally, several prominent physicians and philosophers endorsed his technique in 1930, and his popularity skyrocketed. With subsequent publications and growing popular support, he continued to teach his technique until his death in 1955 at the age of eighty-seven; the technique continues to be taught today throughout the United States and Europe.

What the Technique Is

What began as Alexander's efforts to solve his voice problem evolved over a ten-year period to entail an awareness of the way he abused his own body and the way his body related to his mind. The resulting Alexander Technique relies on seven basic principles:[1]

- We must be completely aware of our bodies and how they function; without this kind of awareness, we cannot make changes to improve our condition.
- Muscle movement is not simple reflex. The muscles actually begin to move in response to mental action: in other words, the second you *think* about moving a muscle, the muscle begins to move.
- You might be hurting yourself without even knowing it: the posture that seems right, the posture you have been taught to maintain, may not be correct.
- Habits are usually not reflexes—most of them are learned and can be changed.
- The body is not made up of a group of separate parts. What happens to one part of your body affects the entire body.
- You can exert conscious control over your habits.
- You can set goals to change your habits, but success is dependent on concentrating on the process, not the goal itself.

Learning the Alexander Technique

Unfortunately, the Alexander Technique cannot be self-taught. Proponents insist that bad posture and bad habits are learned early in life, that they become firmly embedded throughout life, and that only time and persistence from qualified instructors can effect a change.

The technique is not a simple set of exercises. It encompasses instructions on going about all of your activities: reading, writing, walking, sitting, lifting, carrying, even avoiding accidents. The technique is said to be relatively difficult to learn; at least thirty individual lessons are needed from a teacher who helps you connect mental and physical activity and convinces you that you can make conscious choices about how your body functions.

Proponents claim that once you learn and practice the Alexander Technique, you can function at a much higher level than was previously possible.

AUTOGENIC TRAINING

Autogenic training, which employs both hypnosis and biofeedback, was developed by Johannes Schultz in Berlin, Germany, in the 1930s. Designed as a form of medical therapy to normalize mental and physical functioning, autogenic training influences the kind of body function that we do not usually control consciously. Proponents of autogenic training claim that with proper training you can learn to exert control over subconscious and involuntary processes and reduce and control stress, fatigue, and tension.

The premise of autogenic training is that the body will naturally balance itself when directed into a state of relaxation—a state that not only produces self-regulation but promotes self-discovery and awareness.

Practicing Autogenic Training

Autogenic training involves specialized skills and should be undertaken only with the strict supervision of professionals. It should not be attempted on your own without training and supervision.

To practice autogenic training, you must be completely relaxed; lie or sit down, and close your eyes. It can even be done in a noisy place: with the right concentration and training you can practice in a doctor's waiting room, in a busy office, or even on a city bus. What you are aiming for is a condition called *passive concentration* in which you concentrate on one part of your body at a time. You will repeat a phrase several times, and then concentrate on how that phrase has made you feel. To be effective, autogenic training should be practiced twice a day for twenty minutes at a time; you can also resort to it, claim advocates, whenever you need to be calmed or energized.[2]

Start by creating a mood of peace and relaxation. For beginners, advocates advise lying on the floor. You then need to rehearse the following conditions:

1. *Warm.* Say to yourself, "My right arm is warm." Repeat this several times; then move to other parts of your body (such as your left arm, your right leg, and so on). Concentrate on the warmth you have generated.

2. *Heaviness.* Again, select a part of your body, such as your left leg, and repeat the phrase: "My left leg is heavy." Repeat until you feel heaviness, and then move on to other parts of the body.

3. *Calm heartbeat.* Repeat to yourself, "My heartbeat is calm and regular." Concentrate on feeling and controlling your heartbeat. If you begin to experience discomfort, stop this step immediately, and move on to the next step.

4. *Regular breathing.* To further promote relaxation, repeat the phrase, "My breathing is calm and regular." Continue until you are breathing slowly and deeply and until you feel totally relaxed.

5. *Warmth.* Again, you want to create warmth—this time in the solar plexis, or abdominal area. There is an important disclaimer here: *never* try for warmth in the abdominal area if you have suffered abdominal or digestive problems that could result in bleeding from any abdominal organ. This fifth step, say advocates, should be done only under medical supervision. If you have your doctor's okay, repeat the phrase, "My solar plexis is warm." Concentrate on the sensations you feel.

6. *Coolness.* To combine relaxation with awareness, repeat the phrase, "My forehead is cool."

7. *Alertness.* To end your practice, repeat the phrase, "I am refreshed and alert."

At first, say advocates, you probably will not feel much, but, with practice, you will genuinely be able to muster up warmth, coolness, heaviness, and relaxation as you mentally attempt to control those sensations. Proponents suggest keeping a journal of your progress. Try doing only one or two of the steps during short exercise times, but run through all seven twice a day until you have them mastered.

Autogenic Discharge

Advocates report an unusual side effect of autogenic training called *autogenic discharge*. Apparently these discharges are the body's way of getting rid of previously repressed emotional or traumatic experiences.[3] A woman who suffered a crushing knee injury in an automobile accident twenty years earlier may suddenly feel pain in her knees. Other manifestations of discharge include tears, muscle twitching, jerking of the limbs, and a sensation of floating.

Other Applications

Advocates explain that autogenic training, once mastered, can be used for organs other than those specified in the seven basic steps. A practitioner can try to promote warmth, relaxation, and heaviness, in organs or systems not included in the original exercises, for example the sinuses or the chest.

Intentional formulas may also be used—brief, clear, positive self-suggestions directed toward specific changes or specific behavior. Such a formula might be used, for example, to enhance athletic performance during a football game.[4]

The autogenic state can be deepened by using more advanced techniques of meditation; this deeper meditation, explained more fully later in this section, can be induced by visualizing colors and objects, by contemplating concepts, by evoking specific feelings, or by asking questions of the inner self.

Proponents of autogenic training believe the procedure can balance and harmonize the self; release more creative function; cause psychological shifts that enhance the individual positively; regulate habits, such as smoking and alcohol abuse; and cause self-exploration and direction of the body and mind.

BREATHING THERAPY

Advocates of breathing therapy maintain that every emotion we feel is linked to the way we breathe and that proper breathing charges the body with vitality, facilitates health in body tissues, and leads to sharpened mental ability because the brain is properly oxygenated.

Special breathing techniques aimed at disease treatment and prevention were first used by the Orientals and later by the Indian yogis, who developed breathing exercises designed to treat afflictions in various parts of the body. Kept alive through the centuries, the theory of correct breathing involves using the shoulders, chest, and abdomen. Proponents instruct that all breathing—except in cases of real oxygen starvation—must be done through the nose, *not* the mouth.[5]

Why the Nose?

To understand breathing therapy, it is critical to learn the anatomy of the major structure involved: the nose. The nose is the narrowest entrance to the respiratory system, and many probably breathe through their mouths because it is easier: the nose presents much more resistance to air flow, and it takes approximately twice as much work to pull air in through the nose as through the mouth—a mammoth task when you consider that you breathe an average of sixteen times a minute.[6] However, proponents of breathing therapy list thirty important functions performed by the nose—such as registering smell, trapping foreign particles, filtering the air, creating mucus, moisturizing the airflow, and warming the air in preparation for its journey to the lungs—as reason enough to make the effort.

Benefits of Proper Breathing

Breathing therapy advocates cite a number of benefits of breathing properly—deeply, through the nose. Among them are both physical and mental advantages, some of which are immediately apparent.

Because deep breathing quiets the sympathetic nervous system, proponents of breathing therapy prescribe it as a way of relieving stress. To practice, sit in a comfortable position, and concentrate on relaxing all the muscles in your body. Become acutely aware of the process as you breathe deeply through your nose, silently repeating the word "one" each time you exhale. Continue breathing this way, with your eyes closed, for approximately twenty minutes. At the end of the exercise, simply sit and relax for a few minutes before you open your eyes. To be most effective, the exercise should be repeated twice a day.

Advocates of breathing therapy believe that different parts of the brain are stimulated by breathing through each nostril separately, one at a time. They say you can charge your brain to respond with aggressiveness and energy in active situations by breathing through your right nostril and that breathing through your left nostril will enhance passive, quiet experiences.

They cite other mental effects. Breathing through the nose is said to enable you to oxygenate all sections of your brain properly. Some studies have linked mental retardation to mouth breathing: advocates of breathing therapy claim that the upper level of the child's brain never received proper stimulation through nostril breathing, with the result that a disability was incurred. They point out that many mentally retarded people characteristically breathe through open mouths.

Proponents claim that proper breathing can be healing to the emotions and can control impulses of nervousness, jealousy, anger, grief, shyness, hatred, and frustration. The key to emotional control, say practitioners, is slowing the breathing rate and concentrating on deep breathing through the nose.

Physical ailments, too, respond to breathing therapy, say its advocates. Menstrual cramps can be eliminated by deep, slow breathing, and doctors have found a physiological reason: exerting gentle pressure on the tissue inside the nostrils has been shown to make menstrual cramps disappear. Deep breathing through alternate nostrils has relieved the sharp chest pains that signal angina pectoris, a complication of heart disease.

The Right Way to Breathe

According to practitioners, there is a specific proper way to breathe. Paramount in importance is use of the diaphragm—the dome of muscle that separates the chest and abdominal cavities. Forcing the diaphragm down creates a vacuum in the chest cavity that expands the lungs and draws air into them. Pushing the diaphragm up again forces air out of the lungs for exhalation. Breathing with the diaphragm is important, say advocates, because it forces air into the bottom of the lungs, where blood supplies are oxygenated. Breathing with just the chest or shoulders pulls air only into the tops of the lungs, and little blood is oxygenated in return for your efforts. Other important tips: relax and breathe slowly—always through the nose.

POLARITY THERAPY

Polarity therapy is based on the belief that an infinity of universal energy underlies the material world and that man, as part of the infinity of universal energy, is an energy form. Polarity proponents say that energy flows through man's body in channels that are linked together, through all of the vital organs, and through every cell of the body.

The theory is that this energy is polarized in a positive side and a negative side, similar to the yin and the yang in Oriental medicine, and the positive pole is the head, while the negative pole is at the feet.[7]

If there is an alignment and a dynamic balance of physical, mental, emotional, and spiritual elements, there is a corresponding balance of positive, negative, and neutral energy forces which creates a harmony within the individual. Conversely, traumas in life, dietary imbalances, and stress inhibit the free flow of emotions which makes various sets of muscles tighten in patterns which become chronic. This process results in energy blockage and imbalance of the positive, negative, and neutral energy forces.

To increase and balance the vital energy flow, proponents suggest several treatments may be used:

1. *Diet.* Natural foods, fruits, the vegetables are used as main components of the diet to cleanse, purify, build, and maintain the body.

2. *Self-help stretching postures and exercises.* These are mostly yoga postures and other muscle-stretching exercises.

3. *Manipulation.* It is felt that massage can change the energy patterns and polarities in the body because gentle hand contact on specific pressure points can alleviate tension and energy blocks. This massage is similar to the shiatsu massage that is employed as a form of acupuncture. The massage can stimulate the body either in a counterclockwise or clockwise direction, taking into account the polarity of the individual and the condition that must be corrected. The polarity of the person giving the massage must also be considered because it affects the polarity of the receiver. To maintain the proper polarity, for example, it might be necessary to massage the right side of the patient with the right hand.

4. *Attitude change.* The person practicing polarity therapy should have a positive attitude, be open to self-improvement, willing to try to release repressed emotions to reestablish the energy flow, and willing to change attitudinal qualities blocking the free flow of energy.[8]

NOTES

1. Ilana Rubenfeld, "Alexander: The Use of the Self," pp. 222-224 in Leslie J. Kaslof, compiler and editor, *Wholistic Dimensions in Healing: A Resource Guide* (Garden City, New York: Doubleday and Company, Inc., 1978).
2. Vera Fryling, "Autogenic Training," pp. 227-231 in Edward Bauman, Armand Ian Brint, Lorin Piper, and Pamela Amelia Wright, *The Holistic Health Handbook* (Berkeley, California: The AND/OR Press, 1978).
3. Gryling, p. 238; and Norman S. Don, "Four Self-Regulating Therapies in Wholistic Health," p. 234 in Herbert A. Otto and James W. Knight, editors, *Dimensions in Wholistic Healing: New Frontiers in the Treatment of the Whole Person* (Chicago, Illinois: Nelson-Hall, 1979).
4. Fryling, p. 238.
5. M. J. Nightingale, "Air and Light," p. 92 in Ann Hill, editor, *A Visual Encyclopedia of Unconventional Medicine* (New York: Crown Publishers, Inc., 1979).
6. Dina Ingber, "Brain Breathing," *Science Digest,* June 1981, p. 72.
7. Nathaniel Lande, "A Comprehensive Overview of Today's Life-Changing Philosophies," *Mindstyles/Lifestyles,* p. 181; Pierre Pannetier, "Polarity Therapy," p. 216 in Kaslof.
8. Pannetier, p. 216; Alexander Binik, "The Polarity System," pp. 102-106 in Bauman, et. al.

MENTAL
AND SPIRITUAL
REGIMENS

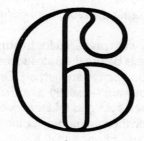

AUTOSUGGESTION

Initially developed by Frenchman Emile Coué in 1885, autosuggestion mimics hypnosis and, in fact, employs hypnosis—even though Coué himself sternly avoided using the word *hypnotism* when referring to his treatments.

Coué's patients were prepared for treatment through a series of hypnotic suggestibility tests before the autosuggestion actually began, to make sure each would be open to suggestion. Once patients were in an altered state of consciousness—exactly like that of hypnotism—they were ordered to close their eyes and told that every word uttered would be permanently etched on their memories. Coué would then give instructions about the mental and physical well-being of each patient.

Coué wrote that constant repetition was necessary to make the ritual work. When the patient's condition began to improve, the length and frequency of sessions were reduced, and they were finally discontinued. The patients themselves played a critical role: every morning before getting out of bed and every night before dropping off to sleep, the patient had to repeat, "Each day, and in every way, I am getting better and better."[1]

Coué himself set the success rate of his treatment at 97 percent.

While the trend was slow to gain momentum at first, by the onset of World War I Coué was treating about 40,000 people each year.

Three basic factors led to the popularity of autosuggestion:

1. First, it seemed to encompass all: it provided help not only for certain organic and physical disorders, but for mental and emotional disorders as well.

2. Second, it was in harmony with the well-known and well-respected work of René Descartes, who had a profound influence on Western thought at about the time Coué was beginning his work. It was Descartes who propagated the philosophy "I think, therefore I am," giving man a hope of gaining power over himself.

3. Finally, the treatment was simple and painless. There were no strenuous regimes for the patient to follow at home, and no bizarre office procedures. All that was required of the patient was repetition of the simple phrase affirming his own well-being.

Ironically, it was the third factor—the profound simplicity of the treatment—that caused autosuggestion to lose popularity as a method of treatment. While a few practitioners still advocate the method, most regard it as too simplistic to be effective as a form of treatment.

BIORHYTHMS

The first physician to suspect that man experiences internal cycles was Viennese Dr. Herman Swoboda, who kept detailed records of patient fevers, heart attacks, asthma attacks, periods of inflammation, and other diseases between 1897 and 1902. Considered the initial proponent of biorhythm, Swoboda noticed as he collected his data that patterns began to emerge, and he postulated that man experiences cycles of twenty-three and twenty-eight days. During his practice, he applied his theory to hundreds of families to explain major life events and to track serious illnesses.[2]

Other physicians practicing during the same period began to draw some of the same conclusions as Swoboda. German physician Dr.

Wilhelm Freeze documented that children developed illnesses at periodic intervals; his work was endorsed by his colleague, Dr. Sigmund Freud. Still another physician carried out experiments with a group of five thousand students; his data served to confirm the presence of the two cycles and to suggest the presence of a third, slightly longer cycle.

Another contemporary of Freud, Dr. Wilhelm Fleiss, was interested in the seemingly periodic affliction of patients with upper respiratory diseases. He launched a research project in which he traced patients' illnesses from birth and inferred the presence of the two shorter cycles.

Despite the mass of research on biorhythms conducted during the nineteenth century, the theory never became popular, probably because the research, with its complicated and involved mathematical formulas, was highly technical and cumbersome. It was simply too much work to figure it out. Research during the past fifty years has made the concept of biorhythms less complicated and easier to understand, and the advent of electronic calculators and computerized printouts has made it possible for the lay public to understand the concept of the three cycles.

The Three Cycles

According to the theory of biorhythms, the birth process is so traumatic that it sets in motion a series of three cycles that continue at regular intervals until death. The three cycles are the physical cycle (twenty-three days long), the emotional cycle (twenty-eight days long), and the intellectual cycle (thirty-three days long). The individual is in a low position for half of each cycle and in a high position during the other half. Crossing over from one to the other creates a critical, or unstable, period during which advocates claim the individual may be more prone to accidents or may exceed his expectations. These critical periods occur in each of the three cycles, so an individual is in a critical period of one cycle or another about one-fifth of the time.

In addition, all living animals and plants have twenty-four-hour cycles or biological clocks that regulate many of their life processes, including human beings. Called *circadian* rhythms, they function almost independently of the surroundings. One of these is the sleep-wakefulness cycle. In an attempt to illustrate the power of this rhythm, researchers have barricaded themselves inside darkened caves without clocks or other indicators of time passage and have found that their patterns of sleep and wakefulness varied little from the normal twenty-four-hour cycle.

Other major rhythms are temperature and performance rhythms. Normally, body temperature varies about two degrees Fahrenheit during the course of a day, and variations in cell division, heart rate rhythms, and other involuntary body processes also occur. Some of these changes are undoubtedly due to the difference in temperature during the day and night; others, claim biorhythm advocates, are part of our natural circadian rhythms. The female menstrual cycle is another biological clock.[3]

The cycles involved in biorhythm allegedly control and influence different life processes. The physical cycle, for instance, determines energy, coordination, and stamina. The emotional cycle governs moods, creativity, and emotional health in general. The intellectual cycle determines the ability to learn, to concentrate, and to make correct judgments. Performance in each of these cycles varies from day to day, of course, even if the same tasks are performed. The difference lies in the individual's point in the cycle.[4]

On positive days, vital energy supply is at its peak, according to biorhythm advocates; on negative days, energy is not as high. The most important days, however, are the critical days, the period when each cycle switches from positive to negative. On those days, an individual is neither up nor down, but in a state of limbo during which proponents believe everyone is more accident- and disease-prone. Sometimes— without apparent rhyme or reason—people may excel beyond their wildest imaginations on critical days.

The concept of biorhythm and critical days has gained wide acceptance throughout the world. Many Japanese taxi and bus companies periodically distribute biorhythm charts to employees in the hope that on critical days drivers will be especially aware of potential accident situations. Apparently the tactic has worked: the Japanese companies have enjoyed a lower accident rate since distributing the charts.

Some airlines have tried periodically distributing biorhythm charts. Some have even carried the concept to the extreme, giving pilots and other employees in important flight positions the day off during a double or triple critical day, a day in which two or three of the cycles switch simultaneously. Critical days for all three cycles fall together in about one out of six critical days—double critical days occur about six times a year, and triple critical days occur about once a year.[5]

It is important to realize that biorhythms do not make things happen. They themselves do not cause disease or accidents. Rather, advocates say, they control vital body energy and indicate times when an individual may be more *susceptible* to illness or accidents.

To calculate biorhythms, consult a biorhythm chart (see Figure 9). They are also available widely from practitioners and others interested in the theory.

HYPNOSIS

Used for centuries as a form of entertainment and as a medical tool, hypnosis was made famous by Sigmund Freud, who used it as an adjunct to his psychiatric practice. Still, the medical profession did not subscribe wholeheartedly to the procedure as a legitimate treatment until 1968, when the American Medical Association approved it as an acceptable mode of treatment. Despite the endorsement, many physicians remain skeptical about hypnosis as a part of conventional medical practice.

A self-induced state of relaxation in which the deeper parts of the mind become accessible,[6] hypnosis causes a suspension of the conscious mind and allows the unconscious mind, which seems more amenable to the powers of suggestion, to take over. Hypnosis is the power of suggestion that either places material in the subconscious or brings material out of the subconscious. It also enables the involuntary body functions to be controlled to some extent.

Though hypnosis has traditionally been used to treat a variety of conditions, it is important to remember that it does not heal or cure. It simply causes actions and reactions that may ultimately lead to relief of the condition.

Hypnosis is probably most widely used to treat emotional problems. Under hypnosis, a patient can vividly recall childhood memories, bring to the surface things completely forgotten, and reexperience the feelings associated with these events. If the experiences were traumatic, recalling them can produce an emotional purging, or catharsis, that relieves the emotional problem and enables the patient to reprogram his or her life into more positive channels.

Charting Your Own Biorhythms

Want to chart your own biorhythms? It's easy!

Let's say you were born March 20, 1954, and you want to find out how your three cycles will look in December 1982. The formula you'll use applies to any case, and it's relatively simple:

First, determine the number of days between your date of birth and the first day of the month you're charting. Don't forget to figure in the extra days during leap years. If you were born March 20, 1954, and you were charting December 1982, you would start this way:

28 years of 365 days each	10,220 days
Days from March 20, 1982, up to and including December 1, 1982	256 days
Extra days for 7 leap years	7 days
Total	10,483 days

Now divide your total of 10,483 days by the number of days in each of the three cycles: 33 in the intellectual cycle, 28 in the sensitivity cycle, and 23 in the physical cycle. Each answer will tell you two things: (1) how many complete cycles you have lived through, and (2) how many days will remain in each cycle as of December 1, 1982. For example, if you divided 10,483 days by 28 (the number of days in the sensitivity cycle), you'd arrive at 374. In other words, you would have completed 374 cycles and you would have 11 days remaining in the cycle.

Let's assume you've done all the necessary figuring. Your cycle chart would now look like this:

10,483 ÷ 33 = 317 complete cycles with 22 days remaining
10,483 ÷ 28 = 374 complete cycles with 11 days remaining
10,483 ÷ 23 = 455 complete cycles with 9 days remaining

You would begin the month of December 1982, then, on the 22nd day of your intellectual cycle, the 11th day of your sensitivity cycle, and the 9th day of your physical cycle. Since the cycle begins with its first "plus" day, this is what your chart would look like:

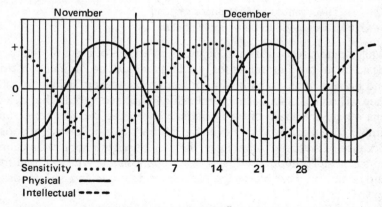

Sensitivity ••••••
Physical ———
Intellectual ————

Your most critical day of the month would be December 3—both your physical and your sensitivity cycles are near the zero line on that day. Your best day would be December 8, when your intellectual and sensitivity cycles are both high. Bad news—during the week of Christmas, December 21 to December 28, all three of your cycles are at rock bottom!

Figure 9

Hypnosis is also commonly used to help patients overcome learned behavior like smoking, overeating, and alcohol abuse. Used in many situations for pain relief, hypnosis has successfully aided women in childbirth and has allowed for painless dentistry. It is beginning to enjoy widespread popularity in the treatment of sexual problems.

Hypnosis has also been used successfully to help people recall needed information: police officials have obtained evidence relating to crimes (a woman under hypnosis, for example, might be able to "see" the license plates on a car that sped away from the scene of a crime, when under normal conditions, she would never be able to remember the plate numbers). Hypnosis can also be used, say advocates, to help an individual discover his real desires or achieve a more positive frame of mind. Hypnosis can also keep goals fresh in the deeper levels of the mind so that the individual is more likely to keep working toward completion of the goal.

People who undergo hypnosis give the following reasons for choosing that form of treatment:[7]

1. They want to take charge of their lives.
2. They want to change certain practices in their lives—especially bad habits.
3. They want to expand their consciousness.
4. They want to achieve peace of mind.
5. It feels good to be under hypnosis.

While some people seek out hypnosis as a form of therapy, many are afraid to submit themselves for fear that they will become unconscious and behave in an embarrassing or inappropriate way. Others fear that they will reveal potentially incriminating information about themselves. Still others are afraid of being dominated by the therapist, and some simply fear that they will never be normal again following hypnosis. Because of these and other fears, the majority of the population cannot be successfully hypnotized: successful hypnosis depends on total trust and relaxation. Fear blocks the process, and no one can be hypnotized against his will.

There are three different degrees of hypnosis:[8]

• *First-degree hypnosis.* Under first-degree hypnosis, the subject hears and remembers everything that goes on while he is in a hypnotic state. First-degree hypnosis is used mainly for treatment of minor problems like general nervousness, minor bad habits, and uncertainties about everyday occurrences.

• *Second-degree hypnosis.* Hypnosis at a much deeper level is commonly used to treat bad habits. Second-degree hypnosis extends further into the unconscious. The subject may not be able to remember everything that is said and done while he is under.

• *Third-degree hypnosis.* The deepest form of hypnosis, third-degree hypnosis is used mainly in the treatment of serious emotional problems and disturbances. The subject does not remember anything that happens.

It takes skill on the part of both the hypnotist and the subject. The subject must be able to concentrate and focus on what the hypnotist is saying, while the hypnotist must be able to induce a state of deep relaxation through simple suggestion.

It is easiest to hypnotize a person who is lying down with his eyes closed. The hypnotist begins the session by suggesting how drowsy and relaxed the subject feels. Heaviness of the eyelids can be induced by having the subject stare at some object until the lids close spontaneously. The hypnotist may then focus attention on the subject's hands and suggests that the hands are light and floating. The hypnotist continues to make these kinds of suggestions until the subject reaches the desired state of suggestibility.

At the end of the session, the hypnotist merely counts backward from five to one, instructing the subject that on the count of one the subject will return to a normal state of consciousness and will feel physically exhilarated.[9]

Every subject is individual: no one person under a hypnotic state will behave the same way as another. Physiological behavior differs from individual to individual: one person may become agitated, while another may remain relaxed and calm.

MEDITATION

Meditation seeks to achieve self-awareness and awareness of the relationship to the environment—both internal and external. During meditation, thinking is separated from perceiving so the individual can stand apart from the emotional self. According to advocates, the practice of meditation renders practitioners more God-conscious and more amenable to the godly qualities of living.

Meditation has been practiced for centuries and is still a vital part of many Oriental, Asian, and Indian philosophies and religions. Buddhists use meditation to purify the mind and gain insight. In the West, meditation is usually used to bring new perceptions and awareness; to relax and heal the body; to make an individual more mentally efficient, more intuitive, and more creative; and to enable an individual to become a more balanced, integrated, and harmonious personality.[10]

Because meditation enables one to achieve a relaxed body state and a quiet mind while maintaining alert wakefulness, some researchers feel that it has better effects on the body and mind than sleeping does.

It can be done at any time, in any environment, but it is best accomplished while sitting in a comfortable position with the eyes closed. Practitioners consciously relax all of the muscle groups—the feet, legs, stomach, chest, arms, neck, face, jaws, and mouth—because decreased muscle tone promotes the meditative state.

The individual must also maintain a passive mental attitude and not try consciously to achieve anything through meditation, as forcing thoughts is believed to make one dwell on himself or herself or prevent the meditating state altogether. Meditating is not designed to prevent all conscious thoughts, but to avoid the continuity of thoughts.

There are many ways of inducing a state of meditation, and most of the methods involve increasing awareness by focusing on the internal environment or some specific aspect of feeling, a thought, a physical process, or a sound. Alternatively, the attention may be directed to an external element of the environment that will remain constant, such as an object, a loved one, a physical activity like a movement of the hand, or the repetition of a phrase or word. This attention to a specific thing causes the separation of the thinking and perceiving systems and enables the individual to free himself.[11]

Breathing may also be the focus. The practitioner can say "one" at each exhalation and exhale twice after each inhalation.

After the meditating period is over, the individual should bring himself back to physical reality and away from the self slowly by leaning over, shaking the hands, perhaps touching the feet. Ideally meditating is done for a period of ten to twenty minutes twice a day to increase the state of total health and well-being.[12]

Proponents of meditation say this practice has many beneficial effects on the body, including slowing the heart rate, lowering the blood pressure, and decreasing the body's need for oxygen. It is said to ease muscle tension and reduce the level of excitation of the nervous system. Further, those who subscribe to the practice of meditation indicate that it has many long-term effects, such as decreasing anxiety, depression, and emotional disturbances; increasing creativity, self-reliance, memory, and perception; increasing reaction time, interaction with the environment, and perceptual-motor performance; and decreasing the need for use of over-the-counter and prescription drugs. Many indicate that meditation helps treat stress-related illnesses such as migraine headaches, spastic colon, and menstrual pain.[13]

PRIMAL THERAPIES

The primal therapies are an outgrowth of a number of different therapies, such as child analysis, psychoanalysis, character analysis, and gestalt therapy, and they attempt to draw people back in time to an initial experience (such as birth or circumcision) to unblock repressed emotions.

The first to experiment with primal therapies was Sigmund Freud, who initially used the term "primal" in 1897. By 1895 Freud had developed many of the concepts he later used in his research but had not labeled them primal concepts. His work with primal concepts is considered by some to be his most outstanding contribution to the field of psychoanalysis.[14]

While psychoanalysts used many of Freud's philosophies through succeeding decades, it was not until 1965 that advocates began to claim that the release of primal processes is a natural self-healing process. This deep delving into the subject's subconscious often releases intense anger, pain, or fear, so primal therapies constitute the most difficult form of psychoanalysis for both analyst and patient. An estimated half of those who began practicing it have since stopped.

RELAXATION THERAPY

In ancient times, the challenges of nature, animals, or other men often made it imperative for primitive man to mobilize all his body energy and faculties to preserve his life. He responded to dangerous situations with a rise in blood pressure, an increase in metabolism, stepped up breathing, and an increase in the blood pumped to the muscles. These body responses still enable man to prepare for fight or flight, though men of today are not subject to the same life-threatening situations. Indeed, people today often experience tension at such a low level of consciousness that they are not even aware they are experiencing stress and taxing the body systems. Because research has shown that tension is abnormal and detrimental to health, much study has been done on relaxation and relaxation techniques. According to Edmond Jacobson, "The purpose of relaxation is to do away with certain activities that place undue tax upon the organism."[15] Most of the techniques involve retraining the muscles of the body to get rid of hidden, underlying tension. Like biofeedback, relaxation techniques seek to teach the individual to recognize even the slight tensions that usually go undetected.

The relaxation response is a restorative process which reverses the effects of the fight or flight response. A comparison of the two shows how the relaxation response may have long-term benefits to health.

Fight or Flight Response	Relaxation Response
Increased sympathetic nervous system activity	Decreased sympathetic nervous system activity
Increased body metabolism	Decreased body metabolism
Increased breathing rate	Decreased breathing rate
Increased heart rate and blood pressure	Decreased heart rate and blood pressure[16]
Increase of blood flow to the muscles	

One of the primary tools for instituting the relaxation response is deep breathing, as tension creates breathing abnormalities which increase tension. People under tension tend to breathe with short, shallow breaths which tend to be thoracic—that is, to use mostly the chest muscles. Thoracic breathing does not allow the lungs to fill completely nor enable the lungs to empty entirely. The stale air is not completely expelled upon exhalation, and the oxygen-carbon dioxide exchange in the tissues is incomplete. This brings about an accumulation of waste products in the tissues which increases tension.

Breathing completely reduces tension. The following technique for correct breathing should be undertaken at least twice a day.

1. Place the hands on the abdomen just below the navel, with the fingertips touching.
2. Breathe through the nose. Mouth breathing is a sign of tension.
3. Inhale slowly. Push the abdomen out so that the fingertips separate.
4. Keep the back straight. This will help the lungs fill and empty fully.
5. Continue to expand the chest and abdomen even after you think you have inhaled deeply.
6. Slightly contract the abdomen and raise the shoulders and collarbone.
7. Hold the breath for five seconds.
8. Slowly exhale from the nose and draw in the abdomen.
9. Let all of the air empty out of the lungs by exhaling more deeply than usual. Hold your breath a second or two before you start inhaling again.[17]

Abdominal breathing brings a measure of relaxation, but there are four other essential elements in achieving relaxation:

- A quiet environment with a minimum of distractions.
- A passive attitude devoid of thoughts about environmental factors.
- A comfortable position.
- Repetition of some mental device. A prayer, a sound, or a phrase may help in obtaining relaxation, as it helps in meditation.[18]

Many favor a sitting position on the edge of a straight-backed chair, with the thighs and the buttocks on the chair, the arms hanging at the sides. The emphasis of this posture is on balance, and there are several exercises to find the points of best balance. First, slowly slide the feet back and forth to find a point of balance where the feet are flat on the floor. The knees should fall open naturally when this point is reached. Make sure that the back is upright and erect. With eyes half-closed, move forward until the lower back muscles pull. Then lean back until the abdominal muscles begin to pull. Move back and forth very slowly until there is no longer any pulling on either set of muscles. Next, still keeping the eyes half-closed, let the head roll forward until the muscles in the back of the neck pull. Let the head move backward until the same pulling occurs on the muscles in the front of the neck. Slowly move the head back and forward until there is no pulling on either set of muscles. Then imagine there is a string running from the top of the head to the ceiling, pulling your body straight up. Straighten the back, and imagine this pulling. Then imagine that the string is cut. The head should be down at this point. Make the left hand (which should originally be in your lap) flop down at your side. Repeat this procedure with the right hand. Repeat these phrases silently three times: "My left arm is heavy and warm. My forehead is cool. My right arm is heavy and warm." Take a deep breath. Bring the hands to the chest, exhale, open your eyes, stretch your limbs. This sequence achieves the best results if it is repeated three times a day.[19]

Relaxation can also be achieved in a prone position. Loosen your clothing, and lie down on a comfortable surface. Do not fold your arms or cross your legs. Keep arms at your sides, the palms down, a few inches from your body. Let your weight sink into the surface upon which you are lying. A bed may be best for this purpose. Imagine that your body is very loose. Slowly stiffen the muscles in both of your arms without moving them or clenching your fists. Hold this position for ten seconds. Then try to stiffen the muscles even more, and hold this position for another ten seconds. While you are stiffening these muscles, take note of how the tension in your arms feels so you will be better able to recognize tension and stiffness on subsequent occasions. Relax your arms gradually so that the stiffness becomes less intense. Rest your arms for one to two minutes. Repeat the whole process again, but this time, let your arms relax more than you did before, past the point of what you would consider to be normal relaxation. The repetition of the process will more forcefully bring to your mind the difference between tension and relaxation. Use this whole process to tense and relax the other muscle groups of the body such as the legs, abdomen, chest, and face. Do not rush these exercises. Forty-five minutes should be an average time for performance.[20]

Many individuals find that self-massage is helpful in promoting the relaxation response. The technique that follows is a suggestion. Note that you should not apply too much pressure to the body. If too much pressure is applied, the muscles will become tense and the purpose will be defeated.

Start at the top of the head. Move the palms and fingertips in a slow, circular motion. The hands should be pressed firmly enough to relieve tension that may have accumulated in the muscles of the forehead and the top of the head. Move the hands forward over the forehead and face and down over the neck and chest, stopping at about the level of the heart. If any place feels especially tense, stop at that place and apply some extra massage. Return the hands to the top of the head. Move down the back of the head, taking time to massage the neck and shoulders. On these areas, you may have to press more deeply, using a rotating motion. When you get to the shoulders, you should use the right hand to massage the left shoulder and the left hand to massage the right shoulder.

Next, grasp the fingertips of the left with the right hand. Move up the back of the left hand and up onto the arm with your right thumb on the underside of the arm and your fingertips on top of the arm. Move your massaging hand up to the left shoulder. Come down the left side of the chest to the level of the heart. Repeat the entire exercise with the fingertips of the right hand beneath the left arm and the thumb on top of the left arm. When you have finished this entire procedure, use the left hand to massage the right hand, arm, and shoulder. Then, with the hands on the abdomen and the fingertips touching below the navel, massage the abdomen and move up from there to the lower chest.

Once you have done this, place the hands on the lower back with the fingertips joined at the coccyx. Massage the lower back deeply with the fingertips. This is a place where much tension is generally felt. Next, grasp the left toes with both hands (the left hand should be on top and the right hand underneath). Apply a good, firm massage to the foot. Press deeply, using the knuckles if necessary. Move up the left leg over the ankles and calves. Continue up the knee and thigh. Repeat this procedure with the right foot. Bedtime is a good time, say advocates, for performing this procedure. Serious relaxation therapy should be done at least once each day.[21]

Relaxation techniques have been successful, say advocates, in relieving conditions like anxiety, high blood pressure, insomnia, colitis, headaches, and other abnormalities usually associated with or caused by tension.

YOGA

Therapeutic yoga was originally used to maintain a healthy mind in a healthy body, but its continuing and expanding use has led to widespread consideration of yoga as a healing technique.[22] During the six thousand years of its known existence, yoga has evolved as a philosophy embracing every aspect of life: physical, emotional, mental, and spiritual. The major philosophies of yoga were developed and published in texts in India beginning in 300 B.C., and yoga came to the West about a century ago with soldiers from India.

The variety of yoga techniques for breathing and positioning the body are designed to improve agility, both mental and physical, and to reduce tension by allowing the body to relax. Yoga proponents maintain that the answer to real happiness is a state of inner tranquility and balance, inner peace and harmony. To achieve this state, it is necessary to dispel the tension that accumulates from the early part of life onward because of the imbalance between the individual and life itself. This continuous tension is a major cause of many maladies, illnesses, and problems, and yoga advocates believe that a majority of physical ills come from mental disease and tension.[23]

As an individual becomes relaxed, meditation is a natural next step, and yoga enthusiasts typically become deep thinkers. While yoga concentrates initially on physical aspects of relaxation, the yoga therapists also work to improve attitudes, diet, posture, emotional attitudes, and spiritual problems. As Theodosia Gardner explains, "Basically, yoga teaches that a healthy person is a harmoniously integrated unit of body, mind, and spirit. Therefore, good health requires a simple, natural diet, exercise in fresh air, a serene and untroubled mind, and a spirit full of awareness that man's deepest and highest self can be recognized as identical with the spirit of God. The law of yoga is the law of life."[24] Thus, yoga embraces every aspect of human life and serves as a system of self-improvement. It is interesting to note that there are different types of yoga to treat whatever aspect of life needs to be remedied or improved. There are emotional, spiritual, mental, physical, and social responsibilities yogas.

It is thought that breath control is the key to relaxation. Various breathing techniques, or *asanas,* are prescribed for healing certain condi-

88

tions, and meditation has been used as a healing force in the treatment of anxiety, depression, nervous debility, and some mental conditions, including schizophrenia. Yogis feel that breathing through the nose controls the flow of *prana*, the vital life force, similar to the ki and ch'i of the Oriental philosophies, into the body. They believe that there is a connection between the function of the brain and breathing, so anger, jealousy, grief, hatred, frustration, and destructive emotions can be controlled by proper breathing. In addition, physical processes can be controlled by proper breathing. The heart slows in response to slower breathing, and this eventually helps to decrease tension.

Like relaxation, yoga maintains that abdominal breathing, using the muscles of the abdomen and the diaphragm, is correct. This breathing enables the lungs to completely fill during inhalation and helps them to empty completely during exhalation so that the amount of residual air is kept to a minimum.

To learn to breathe properly, you might practice the following exercises, which are almost identical to those you learned in the area of meditation. Lie down and place the hands on the abdomen below the navel. The fingertips should touch. Inhale and let the abdomen swell out. You should notice that the fingertips move apart. Exhale through the nose, and at the same time, draw in the fingertips. After exhalation, the stomach should be sucked in to complete the exhalation process.[25]

The three main practices in yoga exercises are the *kriyas,* or cleansing, which includes cleansing the nasal passages with cotton, water, or a rubber tube and forceful expulsion of air from the lungs, bringing with it mucous and other secretions; the *asanas,* postures that accompany breathing techniques, including the well-known corpse posture; and the *pranayama,* or breath control.

NOTES

1. Peter Blythe, "Auto-Suggestion," pp. 186-187 in Ann Hill, editor, *A Visual Encyclopedia of Unconventional Medicine* (New York: Crown Publishers, Inc., 1979).
2. Bernard Gittleson, "Biorhythms," pp. 158-160 in Leslie J. Kaslof, compiler and editor, *Wholistic Dimensions in Healing: A Resource Guide* (Garden City, New York: Doubleday and Company, Inc., 1978).

3. John D. Palmer, "Human Rhythms," *BioScience,* February 1977, p. 93.
4. Michael McDonald, "Biorhythms," p. 52 in Hill.
5. Jean McKenzie, "How Biorhythms Affect Your Life," *Science Digest,* August 1977, p. 18.
6. R. K. Brian, "Hypnotherapy," p. 122 in Malcolm Hulke, editor, *The Encyclopedia of Alternative Medicine and Self-Help* (New York: Schocken Books, 1979).
7. Freda Morris, "Does a Hypnotist Have to Be a Svengali?" p. 241 in Edward Bauman, Armand Ian Brint, Lorin Piper, and Pamela Amelia Wright, *The Holistic Health Handbook* (Berkeley, California: The AND/OR Press, 1978).
8. Hans Holzer, *Beyond Medicine* (New York: Ballantine Books, 1977), pp. 153-154.
9. Morris, pp. 243-244.
10. E. Signy Knutsen, "The Meaning of Meditation," p. 254 in Bauman, et. al.
11. Ibid.
12. Ibid., p. 255.
13. Knutsen, p. 255; and Philip Goldberg, *Executive Health* (New York: McGraw-Hill Publishing Company, 1978), p. 69.
14. William Swartley, "The New Primal Therapies," pp. 208-210 in Hill.
15. Edmund Jacobson, *Progressive Relaxation* (Chicago, Illinois: University of Chicago Press, 1938).
16. Herbert Benson, "The Relaxation Response: Techniques and Clinical Applications," p. 335 in David S. Sobel, editor, *Ways of Health* (New York: Harcourt Brace Jovanovich, 1979).
17. Goldberg, pp. 201-202.
18. Nathaniel Lande, "A Comprehensive Overview of Today's Life-Changing Philosophies," *Mindstyles/Lifestyles,* p. 183.
19. "Tools for Transformation," *New Realities,* p. 44.
20. Goldberg, p. 204.
21. Ibid., pp. 202-203.
22. Vivian Worthington, "Yoga," p. 221 in Hill.
23. Swami Karmananda (Michael Volin), "Breathing to Relax," *New Realities,* April 1979, p. 57.
24. Theodosia Gardner, "Yoga Therapy," p. 538 in Mark Bricklin, editor, *The Practical Encyclopedia of Natural Healing* (Emmaus, Pennsylvania: Rodale Press, Inc., 1976.)
25. Karmananda, p. 58.

HEALING
SUBSTANCES

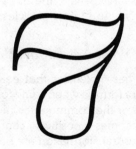

AERION THERAPY

Each of us breathes in and out approximately 10,000 liters of air every twenty-four hours just to survive—and the air we breathe is composed of electrically charged oxygen and water particles called *air ions*.

What Are Air Ions?

Air ions are clusters of gas molecules that bear either a positive or a negative charge. They are formed when some form of energy—such as a cosmic ray—strikes one of the common gas molecules. That molecule loses an electron and becomes a positively charged ion. Other forms of energy that can cause this transformation are present in many everyday situations: the friction that develops when wind whips across the land, when radioactive elements are present in the soil, or when water molecules are pounded by the surf onto the surface of craggy rocks.[1]

Of course, the ion does not stay positively charged for long: in an atmosphere that consists of rapidly colliding ions, the positive ion quickly encounters a neutral ion. The chemistry is again changed, and the ion that results is a negative ion. The incredible collision rate guarantees that the charge-transfer process is a continuous one, resulting in small, medium, and large air ions; the positive ions have a slight edge in numbers.[2] Fresh, unpolluted air contains anywhere from 1,000 to 4,000 ions per cubic centimeter.[3] The picture is vastly different in polluted urban areas: smoking, synthetic fibers, asphalt and concrete, central heating and air conditioning, and air pollutants all inhibit ion exchange. The air in a typical office at the end of the work day may contain as few as 50 ions per cubic centimeter—as little as 2 percent of that found in fresh, unpolluted air.[4]

What Do Ions Do?

What is the importance of the ion concentration in the air?

Apparently, negative ion molecules are important to the growth and vitality of all kinds of plant and animal life—including human growth and development.

Small negative air ions seem to have the ability to destroy and inhibit growth of bacteria, fungi, and various molds—including the organisms responsible for cholera and typhoid fever.[5] They also promote plant growth—especially among beans, peas, barley, oats, and lettuce. Animal studies show that negative air ions stimulate the testes, the ovaries, the adrenal glands, and the thyroid gland and enhance the ability of mice to learn maze patterns.

On the opposite side of the coin, positive air ions have lead to increased deaths from bacterial pneumonia and influenza. Air stripped of negative ions causes plant life to droop and eventually die. Human beings who breathe air stripped of negative ions over a long period of time suffer loss of mental and physical efficiency and can develop a wide range of physical symptoms.

Negative ions promote cell respiration. Too rich a concentration of positive ions causes the release of serotonin—with the resulting dryness, burning, and itching of the nose; nasal obstruction; headache; dry throat; difficulty in swallowing; dry lips; dizziness; shortness of breath; and itching of the eyes. The result? People who are prone to develop asthma, rheumatic irritation, migraine headaches, heart problems, female reproductive disorders, and hay fever start to suffer.[6]

The Therapy

Based on the belief that a higher concentration of negative ions might benefit health and growth, a group of advocates began manufacturing and marketing artificial air-ion generators in the 1950s. Some of the machines produced toxic levels of ozone, and some of the manufacturers began making unrealistic claims about the machines—including their ability to cure cancer. As a result, the Food and Drug Administration issued a statement that negated all health claims stemming from artificial air ionization.

Research that has been conducted since the initial introduction of the ionizers has substantiated some of the claims of the original manufacturers, indicating that ionization may have some benefit in the treatment of certain disorders, such as hay fever and migraine headache.

Advocates claim that only about 30 percent of the population actually needs increased negative ionization, and that an additional 30 percent would simply "feel better." They insist that while 40 percent of the population would notice no change in physical condition, the increase in negative ions would do them no harm.[7]

Proponents advocate the use of artificial negative ionizers for the following conditions:

• *Burns*. Advocates claim that ionizing can reduce the chance of infection and the need for skin grafting in serious burns. When skin grafting is necessary, ionizing can reduce the chance of bacterial infection, according to proponents.

• *Claustrophobia*. Proponents claim that ionization can reduce the effects of claustrophobia—an oppressive feeling of being trapped or shut in—with benefits for workers in small rooms or poorly ventilated areas.

• *Stress*. According to advocates, much of the effect of stress is caused by excess serotonin, and 50 percent of those suffering the deleterious effects of stress, can be relieved by ionization.

• *Victims who suffer from changes in the weather*. Proponents claim that ionization can alleviate symptoms of people who suffer from weather changes—symptoms that include breathing difficulty, asthma, stuffy or runny nose, heart pains, insomnia, irritability, and swelling or pain in the joints.

AROMATHERAPY

Aromatherapy dates back some five thousand years to the ancient Egyptians, who used the scents of aromatic oils such as eucalyptus, lavendar, and clove to treat skin disorders. However, it was not known by that label until the 1930s, when French chemist Rene Maurice Gattefosse discovered that the essential oils used for cosmetic purposes also had medical applications.

Early efforts at aromatherapy included the use of essential oils as antibiotic agents, and most of them were successful antibacterial agents in the treatment of skin infections. With the development of chemical antibiotics, the science of aromatherapy lost interest and support. Advocates today claim that while they are not as effective as chemical antibiotics, essential oils do not carry with them the side effects of the chemical drugs.

Some of the earliest and best-known aromatherapy was carried on by one of Gattefosse's colleagues, who began treating skin cancers with lavender oil. He expanded his work to include treatment of facial ulcers and gangrene, which seemed to heal in record time as a result of the oil.[8]

Aromatherapy practitioners administer the oil in a variety of ways. Essential oils are too strong to be used full-strength on the skin, and the most popular method of administration involves dissolving the essential oil in vegetable oil and massaging it into the skin. Since the oils are readily absorbed into the body and circulated through it, some practitioners claim to be able to treat internal disorders with the skin massage. Some practitioners combine some of the oil with sugar and administer the concoction orally; some even instruct the patient to allow the mixture to melt on his tongue. Since the fragrance of the oils seems to be important in treatment, some practitioners spray the oils around the patient with an aerosol can. Still other advocates use the oils in bath water or in creams, gels, ointments, or lotions.

Advocates of aromatherapy claim that the following physical conditions can be treated successfully with essential oils: suppressed physical immunity (chamomile, lavender, bergamot), poor circulation (cinnamon), inflammation (azulene), oily skin (lavender), dry skin (sandalwood), inflamed skin (chamomile), and influenza (eucalyptus). In addition to physical effects, proponents claim that essential oils can treat emotional disorders and prescribe rose oil for jealousy, chamomile for anger, and hyssop for grief.[9]

While advocates require that specific prescriptions be used in treatment, the use of essential oils has recently gained widespread popularity in the beauty and cosmetic industry.

BACH FLOWER REMEDIES

Trained and qualified in London in 1913, Dr. Edward Bach became convinced that treatment should not center on mere symptoms but on the patient himself. After working in several different branches of medicine, he eventually began practicing homeopathic medicine and started preparing medications in the laboratory of the Royal London Homeopathic Hospital. His work there resulted in seven basic concoctions given orally to treat chronic disease.

Then Bach made a surprising discovery: the patients who required the various concoctions did not necessarily share the same physical symptoms but shared the same mental and emotional state. Bach came to believe that certain emotions rendered a patient ill and demanded treatment. He then carried his reasoning a step further: illness was not a strictly physical phenomenon, but a product of the patient's emotional condition. He began prescribing medication based on a patient's emotions, regardless of the physical symptoms the patient demonstrated.

Quite by accident, Bach eventually discovered that he obtained great relief from exposure to flowers—that his frame of mind and temperament could change if he simply held his hand over a flowering plant. Years of research and experimentation led to his science of flower remedies: he maintained that he could use certain flowers to heal some emotional illnesses that, in turn, resulted in physical ailments.

The flowers Bach used were thirty-eight benign wildflowers; all grow above ground in air and sunlight, and all bear their own seeds. The concoctions he developed are prepared in one of two ways:[10]

• *Early-blooming flowers.* The early blooming flowers, usually those on trees, are picked and immediately put in a sterile, covered saucepan. The saucepan is taken quickly to the house, the flowers are covered with water, and the mixture is boiled gently for half an hour. The water is cooled, the flowers removed; the water is then filtered, bottled, and preserved by adding a touch of brandy.

Bach was clear on appropriate dosages: two drops of water were taken from the saucepan and added to a one-ounce bottle nearly filled with water. Thus, a single saucepan full of boiled water provides a generous amount of the remedy.

• *Field flowers.* This preparation takes place in the field where the flowers grow. The heads of the flowers are picked and placed in water in a simple glass bowl; the bowl is left in full sunlight for three hours. The water at last becomes sparkling and filled with tiny bubbles: Bach believed it was because the water drew the life force from the flowers. The flowers are gently lifted out of the water, and the water is bottled and preserved.

To prepare the medicine, two drops of the water is swirled with one ounce of plain water and a few drops of brandy for preservation.

Methods of Administration

The most common method of administering Bach flower remedies is orally: depending on the urgency of the patient's condition, the remedy may be administered as frequently as every few minutes or as infrequently as once or twice a day.

The remedy is most often administered by dissolving a few drops in a little milk or water, but Bach indicated that it could be mixed in any way that is convenient.

An unconscious patient's lips can be moistened frequently with the remedy.

Less frequently, patients may use external application. A few drops of remedy may be dissolved in a small basin of water, and the water may be sponged or bathed over the affected area. This method is effective against local stiffness, pain, or inflammation, according to proponents. Advocates of external application also suggest dissolving a few drops of remedy in a basin of warm water, soaking a cloth in the formula, and applying the cloth to the affected area; the cloth should be moistened with the formula as needed. Proponents also advise using lotion to soothe any resulting external irritation.

Advocates of Bach flower remedies prescribe these medications not for physical symptoms but for the basic emotional conditions that accompany illness—including despair, fear, uncertainty, loneliness, and apathy.

The thirty-eight remedies have been classified into seven groups, according to the emotion they are intended to ease. Proponents claim that the remedies can be used in all cases of emotional disturbance, including terror, shock, panic, and sorrow.

The seven groups, with their remedies, include:

- *Loneliness:* Heather, impatiens, water violet.
- *Despondency or despair:* larch, elm, star of Bethlehem, oak, crabapple, willow, sweet chestnut, pine.
- *Fear:* Red chestnut, rock rose, aspen, mimulus, cherry plum.
- *Uncertainty:* Cerato, gorse, wild oat, hornbeam, gentian, scleranthus.
- *Over-care for the welfare of others:* Rock water, beech, vine, vervain, chicory.
- *Insufficient interest in present circumstances:* White chestnut, chestnut bud, mustard, olive, honeysuckle, wild rose, clematis.
- *Over-sensitivity to influences and ideas:* holly, walnut, agrimony, centaury.

While there is some question about source among proponents of the Bach flower remedies, it may matter where the remedy is concocted: some research indicates that remedies made in the United States may not be as effective as those made in England.

There are detailed instructions for the use of each flower remedy, and instructions are included when the concoction is purchased. While red chestnut, rock rose, aspen, mimulus, and cherry plum are all generally advocated as the remedy "for those who have fear," the specific flower used depends on the specific characteristics of the fear:

- *Red chestnut,* for example, is prescribed for those who have literally stopped worrying about themselves and are engrossed in fear for others, such as a fear that some catastrophe will happen to a loved one.

- *Rock rose* is commonly used in the most difficult situations, often when the patient has lost consciousness. Called *the rescue remedy,* rock rose is used when there appears to be no hope, either because the patient is absolutely terrified or because he has been involved in a serious illness or accident. Other remedies are often used along with rock rose in these instances.

- *Aspen* is used for patients who suffer from vague, unknown fears that cannot be explained or attributed to any known cause. Such patients often have vague feelings that something terrible is about to happen, but they are reluctant to discuss these fears with others because their apprehensions are completely undefined. The vague fears treated with aspen may occur either during the day or at night.

- *Mimulus,* say advocates, is best used to treat a patient who is afraid of "worldly" things—poverty, misfortune, illness and its ensuing pain, accidents, or being alone. Like the patients treated with aspen, these patients most often bear their dread in secret, only reluctantly admitting their terrible fears.

• *Cherry plum* is used to treat a most unique type of fear: the fear of doing something impulsive and immoral.

All the other remedies are broken down into equally detailed sub-categories and specific moods are described, each with a prescribed remedy. The range of moods includes such varied emotions as absorption with memories (treated with honeysuckle), desire to avoid arguments (water violet, centaury, agrimony), religious fears (aspen), greed over the possessions of others (chicory), procrastination (larch, mimulus, scleranthus), and a lack of sympathy for the plight of others (beech, vine). Despondency may be treated by any of eight different remedies, depending on the characteristics of the mood: despondency caused by feelings of inadequacy is treated with elm; by anguish, sweet chestnut; by feelings of uncleanliness, crabapple; by lack of confidence, larch; by self-reproach, pine; by the limitations of illness, oak; by embitterment, willow; and by shock from bad news, with star of Bethlehem.

Proponents say the practitioner must be sufficiently in tune with the patient to distinguish the causes of various moods and to determine the best treatment—usually not a single remedy, but a combination of remedies suited to the various needs of the patient.

COLOR HEALING

The idea of color therapy is an ancient one: it is believed that the brilliant colors adorning Egyptian and Greek temples were chosen deliberately for their effects on the mind and body. Theories of color healing were common in other countries throughout the world as well, including Tibet, where color qualities are still important in meditation, and India, where color therapy is still practiced. The modern pioneer of color therapy was Rudolf Steiner, whose 1921 series of lectures outlined the use of colors in the treatment of various afflictions.

Advocates of color healing believe that color is a "subtle change in atmospheric pressure from dense red to magenta."[11] Color healing relies on the colors of the natural spectrum separated into four groups—red/orange/yellow, green, turquoise/blue/violet, and magenta. Proponents claim that these eight colors correspond to the twenty-four vertebrae of the spinal column and the twelve bones that make up the sacrum and the skull.

Color has application not only in its correspondence with the vertebrae and skull but also in the color aura that is believed to surround everyone. (Kirilian photography has illustrated that aura, a corona-like structure that displays a multitude of colors, flares, flashes, and rays.)

Color itself is not the only element used in color healing. It is supported by form—that is, certain colors are characteristically in harmony with certain forms. Proponents claim that the color blue is supported by horizontal and spherical forms; red is most often associated with vertical and cube shapes. Yellow is most commonly associated with rays and detaching forms.[12]

Color and form are further combined with rhythmic timing. Rhythm, say advocates, tends to increase the harmony that is initiated by color and form. These three elements can create different responses in the individual—responses that include stimulation, relaxation, nourishment, and neutralization. The specific response produced accomplishes the healing process by producing a realignment of the energy force which produces a healthy molecular structure in the cells.

Practitioner Linda Clark uses a procedure called *dowsing* to diagnose conditions that might be amenable to color healing. She fashions a pendulum by attaching a large bead to a string and holds the pendulum while she proceeds down a list of conditions that can be corrected by color healing, using the pendulum to find out which conditions are present. Clark claims that the pendulum will give yes and no answers to questions if the practitioner is attuned to the powers of the technique; a *yes* answer is indicated when the pendulum turns in a counterclockwise direction. According to Clark, the dowsing technique can be used on self, on others who are present, on others who are absent, and on animals who are either absent or present.[13]

Once the ailment is identified, color therapy is initiated. Different colors are used in different formulas to obtain the desired results. In addition to formulas, practitioners use colors in colored fabrics, walls, and illumination, projected by color-rhythm beamers, lamps, color walls, and color composers. Color images can be established for patients through the use of mental image-making, counseling, and guided meditation.

According to advocates, colors can also be projected on a spiritual level to anyone anywhere for the purpose of healing. To accomplish this kind of healing, a state of meditation must be attained.

Proponents of the theory claim that color healing is useful in both the prevention and the treatment of disease.[14]

HEAT THERAPY

Proponents of heat therapy concentrate on the essential function of blood: while it circulates and delivers oxygen and removes wastes from the system, it also acts in a critical capacity to maintain body temperature. Advocates of heat therapy claim that when body temperature is altered, health is jeopardized. The various forms of heat therapy seek to preserve health not only by stabilizing body temperature but also by applying healing and soothing heat to relieve a number of conditions.

Several major forms of heat therapy are practiced today.

Hot Blanket

Advocates claim that obesity, arthritis, and rheumatic conditions can be helped by treatment with a hot blanket. The aim of the treatment is to induce profuse sweating.

The therapy depends on the preferences of the practitioner and on the condition being treated. The mildest form involves wrapping the patient in dry blankets to increase body heat and eliminate heat loss. Hot water bottles are used to increase the temperature of the blanket wrap.

Burying a patient's body in hot sand is sometimes used to achieve the same effect.

A more drastic form of therapy involves wrapping the patient in a plastic sheet and enveloping him in a specially made electric blanket. Practitioners attempt to reduce discomfort by swathing the head and neck with towels that have been dipped in ice water. Many advocates maintain that the cold-towel swathing is essential to prevent overheating of the brain and overheating of the system as a whole; most rely on it when the treatment is of extended duration.

Wax Baths

Particularly beneficial in treating arthritis of the hands and wrists, proponents say, is the wax bath.

Paraffin wax with a low melting point (usually around 115° Fahrenheit or 46° Centigrade) is melted in a thermostatically controlled tank. Care is taken not to heat the wax to a burning point, because at that temperature, wax could cause severe burns. When the wax is melted, the affected body parts (usually the hands and wrists) are repeatedly dipped and withdrawn to allow the wax to solidify. The treatment specifies eight to ten layers. Once the coatings are applied, the hands are wrapped in waxproof paper and draped with a towel for twenty to thirty minutes.

At the end of the treatment the wax is painlessly removed, and the hands and wrists are held under cold running water for one minute.

Since wax catches fire easily if it is heated too high, advocates discourage home use of wax baths. Wax heated at home should be warmed in the top half of a double boiler over low heat until it liquifies.

Radiant Heat

Radiant heat, used to treat obesity and muscular and skeletal complaints, cannot be used by the very young, the elderly, or those with heart disease or high blood pressure because the dry heat used approaching temperatures of 200° Fahrenheit (93° Centigrade) for treatments of about fifteen minutes. Usually the patient lies on a bed directly under the radiant heat housing. Most radiant heat units are tunnel-shaped devices lined with a reflective material which throws out the heat generated by three or four rows of electric lights.

While fifteen-minute treatments are usually tolerable, advocates stress the importance of swathing the head and neck in ice pads or cold towels to prevent overheating and brain injury. Swathing the face and neck also reduces discomfort and helps the patient withstand the treatment.

Infrared Treatment

The long wavelengths of light located at the red end of the spectrum are the infrared light rays, and they are the rays that carry heat.

Practitioners direct infrared rays at various body parts to relieve the symptoms of kidney disease, gallbladder inflammation, arthritis, and rheumatism. By creating a localized blood temperature that exceeds the temperature of a high fever, the infrared rays cause the blood vessels to dilate and step up elimination of toxins and wastes in the body.

Advocates claim that infrared treatment can be used without damage to the body if several guidelines are followed. The infrared light should be at least six inches from the skin surface, and treatments should never last longer than an hour. People with fair skin should use oil or lanolin to protect them from burns. If the face is involved in the therapy, the eyes should be protected.

Sauna Baths

The principle of sauna baths has been widely used throughout the world to promote health; Romans, Russians, Scandinavians, and Indian tribes throughout the United States, Mexico, Canada, and Central and South America all have their own versions of the sauna bath, which is popularly associated with Finland. While some cultures rely on the sauna bath as a meeting place for exchange of ideas and conversation, other cultures limit them to private sessions for the purification of the body through perspiration loss.

Most saunas are small rooms built of wood and equipped with several benches. Heated stones or rocks inside the room provide heat—ideally between 190° Fahrenheit and 200° Fahrenheit. Advocates claim that the most therapeutic sauna should consist of three phases:

• *Dry heat.* A sauna must always begin with a session of dry heat. Indeed, some feature only dry heat. Dry heat induces profuse perspiration, which advocates say cleanse the body and the skin pores of impurities. Most saunas have benches at various heights: those nearest the ceiling provide exposure to the highest temperatures, and those nearest the floor, the coolest.

• *Moist heat.* When water is poured on the heated rocks, the temperature in the sauna may be increased to 289° Fahrenheit without risks to health. Advocates say moist heat is beneficial to the upper respiratory tract and relieves symptoms of arthritis and various skin diseases.

• *Ice water plunge.* A decreased number of practitioners participate in the third stage: briskly massaging the skin to improve skin tone (done with birch branches in true Finnish saunas) and then plunging into ice-cold water to close pores and rejuvenate the entire system.

While saunas kept at a moderate temperature are usually not harmful, they should not be used by victims of high blood pressure, heart disease, or severe inflammation of the eyes or nose.

HERBAL MEDICINE

The science of plant remedies has been practiced throughout history. Traditional herbal medicine probably dates back several thousand years. The earliest written records were found in Egypt, and other records of herbal medicine have been found in China, India, and Assyria. Many of the herbal remedies outlined in the earliest written records are still widely used by practitioners today.

The most comprehensive early classification of herbal remedies was John Parkinson's *Theatrum Botanicum,* a volume published in 1640 that contains descriptions of more than 3,800 plants and groups them according to their medicinal properties. Contemporary writers have further classified herbs by their main constituents and their pharmacological actions, but volumes as recent as 1977 have built on the classification system started by Parkinson.

Depending on the herb and on the intended treatment, parts of the plant may be used singly or in combination with other parts. Some small herbs are used whole. Generally, practitioners use the seed, fruit, flower, leaf, stem, root, bark, or wood of herbs in preparing remedies.

The skilled herbalist can prepare herbal remedies in any of a number of forms. Probably the most common is the infusion: the fresh herb is boiled, and the water is strained and sipped like a tea, usually several times a day. Woody herbs are boiled in a small amount of water for twenty to thirty minutes. Some herbs are dried, cut, and powdered before being made into remedies.

One of the most common forms of herbal remedy is the tincture: one part of the herb is mixed with five parts of diluted alcohol. Herbal practitioners also prescribe use of herbs in suppository, inhalant, lotion, tablet, pill, and liquid form.

Herbs used in treatment are collected only in dry weather, and advocates of herbal medicine stress the importance of collecting them before noon, drying them rapidly in warm air, and storing them in airtight containers to avoid deterioration. Properly collected and treated and protected from light, most herbs will last for a year without losing potency.

Diseases Treated with Herbal Medicine

Records indicate that herbal medicine has been used to treat almost every medical condition imaginable, and advocates claim that it offers the most complete system of treatment available. Contemporary herbal medicine concentrates on diseases of the blood and the reproductive, pulmonary, digestive, nervous, endocrine, and urinary systems.

Proponents suggest that a combination of herbs be used to treat any single condition because in most cases if one herb is not effective, another will be. They also entreat patients to seek help from an herbal practitioner: many conditions treated with herbs are too serious for self-treatment. In addition, people who have not been trained to recognize the various plants and herbs or who have not been educated about their drug properties are strongly urged not to brew their own concoctions. Physicians are seeing an increasing number of patients suffering from the toxic effects of homemade potions. Herbal practitioners located throughout the United States and Europe offer diagnosis, counseling, and administration of medication.

Some commonly treated conditions and the usual herbal remedies include:

- *Colds and influenza:* peppermint, ginger, catnip, yarrow.
- *Insomnia:* passion flower, hops, lime flowers, American valerian.
- *Nausea and vomiting:* chamomile, peppermint, black horehound.
- *Boils and carbuncles:* marshmallow root, slippery elm, thyme, wild indigo, burdock.
- *Constipation:* licorice, dandelion, blackberry bark, senna.
- *Diarrhea:* agrimony, oak bark, spotted cranebill.
- *Menstrual cramps:* marigold, blue cohosh, passion flower, wild lettuce, false unicorn root.
- *Sore throat:* cayenne, raspberry, thyme, poke root, wild indigo.

The recent resurgence of interest in herbal medicine has led to increased research throughout the United States, Europe, Australia, China, India,

Russia, and parts of Africa, as millions of people use plant remedies either singly or in combination with more conventional forms of medicine.

WATER THERAPY

A natural medicine that benefits the entire body, water can be used in many ways without deleterious side effects to help control many conditions from diarrhea to migraine headaches, according to proponents of water therapy.

As a natural element, water can be used to overcome sudden or chronic energy blocks and can restore the normal flow of internal energy. Cold water, for example, can help revitalize the body during sluggish periods, perhaps because cold water corrects the minor dehydration that may cause weak muscle response, say advocates.

Proponents of water therapy ascribe all kinds of healing effects to water, including the ability to stop a cold before it starts, heal a sore throat, generate energy, relieve pain, vanquish nervousness, help induce sleep, inspire alertness, reestablish internal health, and promote the sexual drive.

Water therapy works on the principle of reflex arcs, nerve points on the skin similar to those used in acupuncture and shiatsu. Water applied to the skin stimulates nerve messages that go to other parts of the body for the healing process, say advocates. External application of water can bathe internal organs, eliminate toxins that cause arthritis, remove unoxidized sugar from diabetics, dilute fluids of the body, correct constipation, eliminate wastes, purify cells, flush the system of illness, increase the movement of blood through the lungs, lower fever, and stimulate liver and kidney activity.[15]

Water is used as ice, water, and steam for therapy, and practitioners may use any liquid pressure, from a light stream to a strong jet.

The temperature varies with the therapy to be performed. Cold water is used as a tonic, a depressant, a restorative, a reenergizer, a builder of resistance, a fever reducer, a thirst quencher, a stimulant, a diuretic, an anesthetic, a pain reliever, a constipation reliever, and an eliminator of toxins. Warm water (referred to as *neutral*) is used for sedation, relaxation, and emetic purposes. Hot water is used to sedate, quiet, soothe, depress and deplete body and muscle tone, induce perspiration, and reduce inflammation and pain. Steam is used to increase skin action and create perspiration (which cleanses the body from within), to open pores, and to ease chest congestion.

External application is generally through baths, showers, compresses, packs, water bottles, ice bandages, wrapped ice, and shampoos. In addition, advocates of water therapy advise internal use through drinking, enemas, douches, and nose and ear baths. Drinking water, say advocates, can bathe the internal organs, dilute body fluids, purify the cells, and rid the body of toxins.

Water is not always used alone in water therapy; other chemicals are sometimes added to effect healing. The most common additions include epsom salts, herbs, salt, lemon juice, fruit juice, vinegar, and witch hazel. Advocates of water therapy advise adding oatmeal, salt, apple cider vinegar, sage, nutmeg, rosemary, pine, hayflower, bran, fennel, epsom salts, ginger, sulphur, borax, starch, bicarbonate of soda, dead sea salt, or algemarin to bath water to relieve skin conditions and soothe sore muscles.[16]

NOTES

1. David S. Sobel, "Breathe Negative: The Positive Effects of Negative Ions," *Medical Self-Care,* Spring 1980, p. 28.
2. Albert P. Krueger, "On Air Ions—Your Health, Moods, and Efficiency," *Executive Health,* Volume XVII, Number 2, November 1980.
3. Sobel. p. 28.
4. Sobel, p. 29.
5. Krueger.
6. Felix G. Sulman, "Aeriontherapy," p. 140 in Leslie J. Kaslof, compiler and editor, *Wholistic Dimensions in Healing: A Resource Guide* (Garden City, New York: Doubleday and Company, Inc., 1978).
7. Ibid., pp. 139-140.
8. Robert Tisserand, "Aromatherapy," pp. 124-125 in Ann Hill, editor, *A Visual Encyclopedia of Unconventional Medicine* (New York: Crown Publishers, Inc., 1979).
9. Ibid.
10. Nora Weeks, "Bach Flower Remedies," pp. 122-123 in Hill.

11. Theo Gimbel, "Colour Therapy," p. 218 in Hill.
12. Ibid.
13. Linda Clark, *How to Improve Your Health: The Wholistic Approach* (New Canaan, Connecticut: Keats Publishing, Inc., 1979), pp. 31-36.
14. Gimbel, p. 219; Clark, pp. 36-38.
15. Dian Dincin Buchman, *The Complete Book of Water Therapy* (New York: E. P. Dutton, 1979), p. 16.
16. Ibid., pp. 73-74.

MACHINES
AND INSTRUMENTS

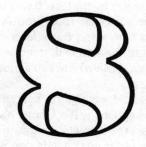

ACUPUNCTURE

Acupuncture, a well-known form of Oriental medicine, was discovered in China thousands of years ago by mistake: it was noted that soldiers who were wounded with arrows often recovered from diseases that had plagued them for years.[1] Imitating the effects of the arrow, Chinese doctors began to puncture the skin with needles at certain points in an effort to determine the relationship between various body points and the organs affected by disease.

The earliest medical writings on acupuncture appeared more than four thousand years ago in the *Nei Ching,* a volume that took more than fifteen hundred years to complete. At first, the acupuncture needles were made of stone quarried from rich jade deposits in the mountains of China; later, Chinese doctors used needles fashioned of bone or bamboo. When metal was discovered, the needles were made of iron, silver, copper, gold, and other alloys; today's needles are made of processed stainless steel. The wide variety of materials used to make acupuncture needles refutes the claim that it is the metal, not the actual needle, that produces effects.

The use of acupuncture as anesthesia began in 1958, when it was first used to relieve postoperative pain. Its effectiveness as a pain reliever led doctors to consider its use as a general anesthesia during surgery, and, later that year, a patient underwent a tonsillectomy with only acupuncture as anesthesia; the patient reported no pain during surgery and no aftereffects of the acupuncture.[2] The next year, in 1959, acupuncture was successfully used as anesthesia in surgery of the brain, chest, limbs, abdomen, and back.

Today more than a million doctors in China rely solely on acupuncture as anesthesia during surgery; about 20 percent of the surgical operations performed in China are performed with no other anesthesia, and many other operations involve a combination of acupuncture and more conventional types of anesthesia. Acupuncture is practiced by more than three million doctors in the Orient. It is used in hospitals in France and Germany and is taught as a medical practice in several universities in Russia. More than 10,000 doctors in the United States have adopted acupuncture as a tool in both diagnosis and therapy.[3]

How Acupuncture Works

The ancient Chinese practitioners identified twenty-six meridians, pathways or channels in the body through which the *ch'i,* the vital energy force, flows.[4] The meridians link a series of points where energy and blood converge; there are eight hundred of these points in the body. Each point or set of points is associated with a specific organ or body function.[5]

According to proponents of the theory, disease results when the flow of ch'i along the meridians is blocked; for a healthy state, the ch'i must flow unobstructed along the meridians. Locating the obstruction and stimulating or relaxing that point with acupuncture makes the pain and/or disease disappear, as the balanced energy flow is restored.

Skilled acupuncturists claim to make their diagnosis by feeling the pulse points along the meridians. Quietness, overactivity, underactivity, hardness, or fullness of the pulse points can indicate an excess or depletion of the energy flow through the meridian. Sensitivity plays an important role, too—practitioners say that when malfunction occurs in a certain organ, the corresponding meridian points will be sensitive when touched.

Once the exact points needing treatment have been located, the acupuncturist inserts a needle into each one; the depth of insertion depends on the extent of the disease and the body system that is being healed. Depending on the treatment needed, the needle may be left in place for only a few seconds or up to a period of several weeks; sometimes the needles are manipulated by hand or by machine once they are inserted. According to those who undergo acupuncture, it is relatively painless: insertion of the needle by a skilled practitioner feels somewhat like a small pinprick followed by a feeling of tingling or pressure.[6] When done correctly, acupuncture usually draws no blood, and the sensation is usually felt for up to half an hour after the needle is removed.

During diagnosis, the skilled acupuncturist can allegedly tell whether there is too much or too little energy flowing through the meridian. The acupuncture needles are inserted and manipulated accordingly: they can stimulate more energy flow or relax the meridian points to decrease and balance the energy flow. According to practitioners, acupuncture done correctly results in a dramatic reduction of disease symptoms and can result in changes in red and white blood cell counts, changes in the body's immune capabilities, changes in the heart rate, and dilation of the breathing passages and the blood vessels. As a result, proponents claim it is effective in the treatment of high blood pressure, depression, anxiety, migraine headache, arthritis, lumbago, digestive tract diseases, fibrositis, rheumatism, dermatitis, eczema, psoriasis, asthma, bronchitis, ulcers, sciatica, neuritis, neuralgia, low back pain, and muscle or skeletal pain.

Most acupuncture in the United States is used for relief of chronic pain. Treatments have been effective in one out of ten patients, and another 15 percent of patients with chronic pain have received partial relief.[7]

Still another application of acupuncture is in disease prevention: skilled acupuncturists should be able to predict the occurrence of disease and prevent it by monitoring the flow of ch'i through the meridians.[8]

Why Acupuncture Works

There are a number of theories as to why acupuncture works. Some believe that it simply stimulates the body's own regenerative powers—the same powers that cause us to flush the eye with tears when a piece of dust is lodged under the eyelid or to cough forcefully when a small piece of food enters the windpipe. Others claim that it increases circulation, always a benefit to health.

Recent research results indicate still another important possibility: that insertion of acupuncture needles stimulates the nerves and causes the brain to release endorphins, painkillers manufactured in the brain that work like morphine.[9]

Finding an Acupuncturist

To find a practicing acupuncturist, learn how your state laws govern the art. Currently, only four states license acupuncture as a separate healing art. In those states—California, Hawaii, Nevada, and New York—practitioners must pass state licensing examinations similar to those administered to medical doctors. In eleven other states, acupuncture is permitted only if the acupuncturist practices under the supervision of a physician. In about half the states, acupuncture can only be practiced by a medical doctor, a chiropractor, a dentist, or a physician's assistant.

According to the American Medical Association, acupuncture is still regarded as an experimental medical procedure. Some insurance companies will pay for acupuncture performed by an acupuncturist if the procedure is legal in the state where it was performed and if the procedure was prescribed by a physician; many other insurance companies will pay for acupuncture if it is performed by a physician. Check your state laws and your insurance company's policies if you are considering treatment.[10]

BIOFEEDBACK

The premise of biofeedback is easily stated: if you can become aware of body functions that you usually are not aware of, you can eventually learn to control those functions.

It has long been believed that man's ability to control and conquer nature could be channeled into the ability to control his own well-being, but as a technique, biofeedback has come into more extensive use only during the past several decades. The modern method was pioneered in the 1960s by San Franciscan Dr. Joe Kamiya, whose original experiments monitored brain activity. Interest in biofeedback blossomed, and research during the last few decades has broadened and refined the practice.

The origins of biofeedback go back to the Indian yogis, who learned to control involuntary body processes like heart rate. British Army doctors who encountered these yogis reported that their success seemed to be a result of long-term practice of certain physical, mental, and emotional disciplines.[11]

Late in the nineteenth century scientists made some of the discoveries that led to postulation of the principles governing biofeedback. Luigi Galvani discovered that frogs' legs twitched when stimulated by electric signals, and he used electric stimulation to cause muscles to move. Later, in 1878, Romain Vigoroux discovered that the electrical resistance of the skin varied with changes in consciousness. Their work led to the development of the sophisticated instruments currently used in biofeedback that measure galvanic skin response and basal skin resistance.

Still a third discovery late in the nineteenth century contributed to the science of biofeedback: British researcher Richard Caton discovered that rabbits and monkeys generate electrical signals and that those signals vary, depending on the amount of stimulation the monkey receives. At the turn of the century Western doctors became increasingly interested in attempts to control bodily functions, an interest that led to the development of autosuggestion. Further research into the electrical activity of the brain and its effects on the body led eventually to the development of biofeedback as a science.

Biofeedback Process

Biofeedback is one means of learning to exert control over involuntary body processes below the level of consciousness that affect overall health. It uses devices to monitor such processes as breathing, heart rate, blood pressure, skin temperature, and muscle tension. According to advocates, if a person is given information about how one of his internal, involuntary systems functions, he can eventually learn to control the activity of that system. Put simply, proponents say the mind cannot direct the body unless it knows what is going on inside the body. Biofeedback gains this information from the body, gives it to the mind, and extends the capabilities of the mind so that both body and mind can be controlled.

Most often, this monitoring is accomplished through the use of visual and auditory monitoring signals—for example, if the patient is trying to control his heart, he is attached to a device that will allow him to hear his heart beat or see the pattern his heartbeat creates on a graph. Advocates claim that if a person can see how fast his heart is beating or hear the beating he can learn to control his heart rate to some extent.

How Control Is Learned

The control of skin temperature is a good illustration of how biofeedback works. Skin temperature is a reflection of the blood flow to an area: as the circulation increases, so does the skin temperature. Circulation and skin temperature can be increased by a number of factors, including exercise, tension, environmental factors, or disease conditions.

For the sake of example, assume that a man is experiencing cool skin because of stress and tension; if he reduces the amount of tension he is subjected to, his skin temperature will warm as a result. To reduce tension—and thereby increase skin temperature—the man might think of a relaxing situation in which he felt comfortable, happy, and tension-free; if he is attached to a monitoring device, he will be able to see a change as he envisions the pleasant scene. His skin temperature will increase.

The goal of biofeedback training is to train an individual to see and hear what is going on and eventually, to discontinue use of the monitors when the individual can sense that he needs to use his biofeedback training. The person trained to increase his skin temperature, for example, will be able to detect even minute drops in his skin temperature without thermometers or monitors and will be able to recreate the pleasant thoughts that brought his skin temperature under control.

Monitoring Involuntary Processes

Four common means are used to monitor involuntary processes:

• *Galvanic skin response.* Electrodes are attached to the fingertips to monitor the electrical activity in the skin.

• *Electroencephalogram.* Electrodes attached to the scalp measure the electrical activity on the brain's cortex. The desired end of biofeedback and other forms of relaxation training is to separate the physical and the mental: to allow an individual to be mentally alert without being physically tense.

- *Electromyograph.* Electrodes attached to the forehead measure muscle tension. The most widely used biofeedback monitoring device, it is the easiest and the quickest means for learning biofeedback control.[12]
- *Skin temperature.* Thermistors attached to the fingertips monitor warmth of the skin.

How Biofeedback Works

There is an important distinction to note: advocates do not claim that biofeedback cures physical ailments. They simply claim that it can motivate the patient to pinpoint the various involuntary processes causing him distress and to formulate his own treatment. Biofeedback proponents claim that the process of biofeedback, if properly exercised, can cause a patient to regard illness as a lesson that will help the individual to reevaluate goals and attitudes, initiate unrealized potential, and improve the quality of life.

Biofeedback's farthest reaching potential probably lies in the relief of tension and anxiety, since tension and its resulting stress are most likely the primary cause of unhealthy involuntary processes. The best results in this area have been achieved when biofeedback has been used to relieve migraine headaches. Other successes have been recorded in the treatment of high blood pressure and spastic colon, both of which are commonly caused by tension and anxiety.

Like many other alternative healing methods, biofeedback is more effective as a means of disease prevention than as a means of disease treatment. Many practitioners strive to help patients control tension and anxiety *before* they result in a disease condition and before patterns of tension are well established in the body.

ELECTROTHERAPY

Electrotherapy—the use of electricity to treat medical disorders—had its formal beginnings with Italian physician Luigi Galvani, who noticed that tiny currents of electricity caused freshly dissected frogs' legs to twitch. That form of electrotherapy now bears his name, Galvanism. Once widely used in the treatment of athletic injuries, it is now typically used only when other forms of electrotherapy have failed.

The use of electricity in the treatment of medical disorders actually began before electricity was harnessed: two thousand years ago the Romans used electric eels to soothe the pain of gout. Throughout the 1800s electricity was used principally to heal broken bones (a use that continues today), but by the end of the century charlatans who devised electrical "appliances" that claimed to do everything from curing cancer to banishing impotence earned electrotherapy a reputation as mere quackery.

Beginning with Galvani's work, however, researchers discovered the vast network of nerves and their influence over muscles, and the effects of electricity over both the nervous and the muscle system led to advances in the treatment of various disorders and diseases.

Electricity is used today in both external and internal applications as a remedy for a number of medical conditions, some of them previously untreatable.

External Applications

One of the earliest applications of electrotherapy—to treat broken bones—is today one of the most common uses of external electrotherapy. Using electromagnetic coils invented by Michael Faraday, early therapists enjoyed a high success rate in both the treatment of fractures and the regeneration of nerve and muscle injuries. Today's electromagnetic coils are encased in plastic pads; some are shaped like ping-pong paddles, while others resemble shin guards. The pads are connected to a pulse generator that plugs into an ordinary wall outlet. The patient does not feel the mild pulsating current that bathes the fracture site, and orthodox medical practitioners report success in about 80 percent of the cases, when the current is used for a period of three to five months, twelve hours a day. (These studies were done on fractures that had totally resisted conventional treatment.)

Proponents of electrotherapy are also using small external units powered by batteries to relieve the pain of muscle injury, usually the sprained ankles and lower-back injury common to athletes. Called *transcutaneous electrical nerve stimulators,* the devices must be used six to eight hours a day to provide relief for aching joints and muscles. They were used by athletes at the 1980 Lake Placid Winter Olympics to ease soreness and stiffness following workouts and competition.

While transcutaneous electrical nerve stimulators are widely used by orthodox practitioners, a version of the therapy called *inferential therapy* is advocated and practiced by unorthodox healers. Instead of a single pulsating current, two separate medium-frequency currents are superimposed at the desired site in the tissues. At the point where the two frequencies meet, they cause a low-frequency pulsation which advocates claim can increase circulation, control pain, and promote movement. Proponents of inferential therapy claim that the higher voltage electric current improves blood and lymph circulation and tones and exercises damaged muscles.

Still higher frequency and voltage is used in sinusoidal current therapy, which was formerly used to stimulate both motor and sensory nerves. Use of sinusoidal therapy has sharply diminished, in part because the skin irritation from the high frequency is difficult to tolerate.

A type of external electrotherapy pioneered in 1934 by Dr. Abraham Ginsberg in New York, high-frequency therapy, is used by advocates to promote deep healing in body tissues. Initially used in the 1940s, high-frequency therapy was a successful means of treating rheumatoid arthritis, bursitis, sinusitis, and many bone and muscle problems, including strains, sprains, and fractures.

According to practitioners, high-frequency therapy can speed healing by as much as 50 percent because of its effects: it sharply reduces pain, disability, and swelling, and eliminates bruising of tissues and tissue swelling caused by water retention in cells. In addition, high-frequency therapy has been used by orthodox physicians to heal bone fractures and to quicken the formation of new skin following burns.

Some practitioners and orthodox physicians agree that high-frequency therapy is the one form of electrotherapy that promotes healing without any kind of tissue damage.

Internal Applications

Widely used in both orthodox and unorthodox medicine, internal applications of electrotherapy continue to be the subject of intensive medical research.

The most famous internal use is the heart pacemaker—the hockey-puck-shaped device implanted under the skin of the abdomen or the chest that delivers tiny electrical impulses to stimulate a regular pattern of activity in the heart muscle. Modern technology has effected some significant changes in pacemakers: batteries, once good for only a year or two, now commonly last ten years or more, and some of the newest models are not much larger than a quarter. Some of the most recent pacemakers come with an external unit that can be reprogrammed to meet the changing needs of the patient.

Even more incredible than the modern pacemakers is a unit called the *automatic implantable defibrillator*. Operating on the same principles as the large external defibrillators, the small implanted unit keeps track of the heartbeat and delivers one high-voltage jolt to the heart muscle if the rhythm becomes irregular. While the jolt may be as high as 700 to 800 volts, practitioners report that the sensation is not painful to the patient.

Internal therapy is also being used to regenerate bone growth. The circuitry is actually dependent on both external and internal units: two wire electrodes are drilled into the broken edges of the bones and connected to a small power pack sealed inside the patient's cast. The power pack is connected to still another unit that is attached to the patient's skin outside the cast. This three-way circuit, both external and internal, allows mobility that is not possible for the patient using the external form of therapy, who must limit motion and keep weight off the affected limb.

Research is currently being conducted on electrodes which, when implanted in the fingers and hand, may allow paralysis victims to regain partial movement of the fingers. Still other research, involving implantation of tiny electrodes along the inner ear, seeks to reverse some kinds of deafness.[13]

Among the most controversial uses of internal electrotherapy is implantation of electrodes in the central gray area of the brain—the area of the brain, it is believed, that triggers the release of endorphins, or natural pain-killers. A handheld device would allow the patient to stimulate pain relief by releasing endorphins and blocking nerve impulses. Used primarily for victims of chronic and terminal pain, the twenty-minute stimulation can provide up to twelve hours of continuous pain relief. The method has also been used by some mentally and emotionally disturbed patients to restore calm, a use that has prompted some opponents to claim that the device could be used to control thoughts or emotions.

LAKHOVSKY OSCILLATORY COILS

Beginning with some of the same philosophies that prompted development of electrotherapy, French engineer Georges Lakhovsky decided that the health and vitality of the human being depended on the proper balance of the oscillating nucleus in each cell in the human body.

In the course of research in the 1920s, Lakhovsky came to feel that the tiny twisted filaments visible in the cell nuclei were capable of receiving and transmitting radiation, and he concluded that disease was nothing more than a disturbance of the oscillating properties of the nuclei.

Working with patients, Lakhovsky tried out his theory. He postulated that by giving cells an electrical jolt, he could induce the diseased cells to oscillate at a different rate, which would restore them to their original rate of oscillation without harming tissues or cells.

Once he became convinced of his theory, he set about developing a device that would enable him to deliver the proper jolt. In 1931 the multiple wave oscillator resulted, and it was readily adopted by a number of French hospitals, where it was used to treat diseases, including cancer. The device was composed of two large coils, one a transmitter and the other a receiver. The area to be treated was placed between the coils, an electromagnetic field was created, and the oscillation allegedly passed through the tissues, restoring them to health. Treatments consisted of several periods of up to fifteen minutes a day.

The original oscillator was incredibly large and bulky and extremely expensive, which limited its usefulness. Continuing research by advocates has resulted in a smaller, less expensive version, known as the Lakhovsky Oscillatory Coils.

MICROWAVE DIATHERMY

Microwaves are a form of electromagnetic radiation used by health practitioners for deep-heating the muscles to increase blood flow. Studies show that microwaves can penetrate approximately two inches below the body surface and can raise the temperature of the muscles to 106° Fahrenheit—enough to dilate the blood vessels that nourish the muscles. The increased blood flow that results, say advocates, provides for a more rapid transfer of nutrients which, in turn, reduces pain and promotes tissue healing.

An additional benefit to the tissues, say researchers, is the accelerated removal of waste—including toxins and bacteria—from the treated area.[14]

The device that produces the microwave radiation is called a *magnetron tube*. It is a high-frequency generator, that converts electrical energy into high-frequency energy. The area of the body to be treated is positioned under an applicator that is connected to the tube with a cable. The applicator is positioned two to six inches from the site of treatment. Most treatment sessions last about twenty minutes. The applicators used are most commonly round, but they vary in size and shape with the area of body being treated.

About 10,000 of the units are currently being used in the United States by physicians, chiropractors, physical therapists, and medical technicians. One of the most common uses is the treatment of athletic injuries, but an estimated 25 million additional treatments are given each year for sinus conditions, eye diseases, dental problems, chronic pelvic inflammations, tendonitis, arthritis, and bursitis.

The advantage of microwave diathermy is that microwaves produce heat only where they are absorbed. They do not heat other tissues of the body, nor do they produce the characteristic physiological effects associated with heat production.

The Food and Drug Administration recently stepped up regulatory control of the microwave equipment used in diathermy, and urged prospective patients to undergo treatment only from an authorized physician.[15] The FDA did not pass judgment on the value of diathermy as a therapy, but the agency did issue certain warnings: microwave diathermy should never be used on patients who are unconscious or on areas of the body where metal is implanted (including metal joints, dental fillings, intrauterine devices, or metal sutures).

Other regulations currently under consideration are aimed at limiting the amount of heat put out by the applicator, limiting the chance of radiation leakage from the equipment, installing safety equipment to shut off the machine in an emergency, and circulating to advocates, physicians, and prospective patients information on the safety and proper use of the equipment.

Usage information is critical, according to FDA officials. Physicians have been instructed to exercise extreme caution when using microwave therapy on the head or in the genital areas and to be aware that damage to the fetus of a pregnant woman could result.

MOXIBUSTION

Moxibustion, a form of acupuncture that uses heat, apparently had its beginnings almost two thousand years ago in China. One early documented report claimed the cure of chronic headaches through the technique of moxibustion.

Moxa cones or moxibustion sticks, made of compacted dried herbs, are placed on the acupuncture point that needs to be stimulated, and the cone or stick is lighted. When the subject feels some pain and heat, or when the stick is burned nearly to the skin, it is removed. The results are similar to those gained from piercing the skin with the acupuncture needle, but the subject feels pleasant warmth at the site. Because the cone is so swiftly removed, pain is rarely felt.

There are some variations on the method. Rarely, the heated end of a moxa stick is applied with the lighted end on the skin surface and removed when the subject feels the warmth. Another method involves the use of a needle that has a cup at one end that is filled with moxa; when the moxa is lighted, the heat runs down the needle to warm and penetrate the acupoint.[16]

NOTES

1. Sidney Rose-Neil, "Acupuncture," p. 56 in Ann Hill, editor, *A Visual Encyclopedia of Unconventional Medicine* (New York, New York: Crown Publishers, Inc., 1979).
2. Rose-Neil, p. 60.
3. Ibid.
4. Rose-Neil, pp. 56-60; Richard Grossman, "Richard's Almanac," *Family Health,* April 1979, p. 52.
5. Rose-Neil, p. 56.

6. "Acupuncture: A Curious Cure That Works," *Changing Times,* November 1980, p. 39.

7. C. Norman Shealy, "Holistic Management of Chronic Pain and Distress," *New Realities,* April 1979, p. 67.

8. David E. Bresler, Richard H. Kroenig, and Michael P. Volen, "Acupuncture in America," in Leslie J. Kaslof, compiler and editor, *Wholistic Dimensions in Healing: A Resource Guide* (Garden City, New York: Doubleday and Company, Inc., 1978), p. 133.

9. "Acupuncture: A Curious Cure That Works," pp. 38-39.

10. Ibid., p. 38.

11. Tim Scully, "Biofeedback and Some of Its Non-Medical Uses," pp. 201-203 in Edward Bauman, Armand Ian Brint, Lorin Piper, and Pamela Amelia Wright. *The Holistic Health Handbook* (Berkeley, California: The AND/OR Press, 1978).

12. Philip Goldberg, *Executive Health* (New York: McGraw-Hill Publishing Company, 1978), pp. 185-186.

13. Dennis Meredith, "Healing with Electricity," *Science Digest,* May 1981, pp. 53-57.

14. James Greene, "Microwave Diathermy: The Invisible Healer," *FDA Consumer,* February 1979, p. 7.

15. Greene, p. 8.

16. The Revolutionary Health Committee of Hunan Province, *A Barefoot Doctor's Manual* (Seattle, Washington: Cloudburst Press, 1977), p. 45; and Sidney Rose-Neil, "Moxibustion," p. 68 in Hill.

APPENDIX: A SUMMARY OF THE THEORIES AND THERAPIES

The chart that follows provides a brief overview of some of the alternative theories and therapies currently being practiced. The theories and therapies, listed in alphabetical order for convenience, are accompanied by brief descriptions, benefits claimed by proponents, and statements concerning validity.

Not every therapy discussed in the text is included in this chart. You'll also find listings of a number of theories and therapies that are not included in the text: instead of merely repeating those theories discussed in the text, this chart is intended to provide smatterings of information on a wide variety of alternative healing practices.

While the validity of some theories and therapies is well-documented and accepted, the validity of others remains in question. Note that a number of theories and therapies are followed by statements such as "Documentation needed," or "Limited scientific evidence available." In such cases, proponents have provided only limited documentation, and you should carefully weigh a decision to pursue practitioners in these therapies.

This chart was developed with the assistance of Laura Lewis.

MEDICAL THEORY, THERAPY OR APPROACH	TECHNIQUE OR PROCEDURE	BENEFIT CLAIMED	VALIDITY
Acupuncture	Needles are inserted at certain points of the body (meridians) where "vital energy" flows	Anesthetic; treats migraines, headaches, ulcers, arthritis, high blood pressure, depression, bronchitis, etc.	Use as anesthetic is fairly well-documented; in some circumstances more research is needed
Air and Light	Expose body to air and light	Beneficial for skin and general health	Accepted practice in some circumstances as long as exposure is not excessive
Applied Kinesiology	There is a relationship between certain muscle groups and organs; muscles are tested for strength and tone, indicating "balance of energy"; if muscles are weak, this indicates that the energy is not balanced, possibly because of diet and/or stress	Indicates status of certain organs or body systems	Limited scientific evidence
Aromatherapy	Fragrant oils applied to skin	Antibacterial agents used to treat gangrene, facial ulcers, and skin cancer	Documentation needed
Autogenic Training	Self-influence upon mental and bodily functions	Assist in dealing with stress, and improve general health	Documentation needed
Autosuggestion	Self-administered suggestions to bring about psychological or physical change without conscious effort	Initiate self-healing	Documentation needed
Bates Method of Eyesight Training	Blink frequently; splash eyes while closed with warm and cold water, change focus from near to far and vice versa	Rests eyes, and aids in circulation, and improves functioning of eye muscles	Documentation needed

MEDICAL THEORY, THERAPY OR APPROACH	TECHNIQUE OR PROCEDURE	BENEFIT CLAIMED	VALIDITY
Biofeedback	Teach person to become aware of disfunctional body organ or system and how to control it	Improve health status	Some successes, further research and documentation needed
Biorhythms (Rhythms of life)	Evaluation of physical and emotional cycles	Relate to behavioral pattern; alert person to deal with energy variations	Documentation needed
Chiropractic	Rapid manual manipulation, especially of the spine; utilizes diagnostic X-ray more than osteopathy	Eliminate back pain; heal diseases and promote good health	Limited scientific documentation
Clay Treatment	Apply clay to skin	Antiseptic and antibiotic properties	Documentation needed
Copper	Wear copper next to the skin (bracelet, rings, or necklaces)	Alleviate pain from rheumatoid arthritis	Documentation needed
Cupping	Heated cup is placed on skin; as it cools, a vacuum is formed	Used to relieve migraines, bronchitis, asthma, boils, arthritis, etc.	Documentation needed
Electrotherapy	Electricity is applied directly to body surfaces	Treats disease, injury, circulation, and speeds up toxic waste removal from inflamed areas	Some success; more documentation needed
Gems (related to Spectrum Colors)	Place gems in living environment or wear next to skin	Therapeutic effects to various body parts, due to different energy levels of the various gems	Documentation needed
Healing	Emotional relationships are established through mind patterns of force; trust and love must be present	Aids in healing	Documentation needed
Heat	Heat application by sauna baths, hot blankets, infrared rays, baths, and so on	Aids skin in waste elimination; relaxes muscles	Documentation needed

Hypnosis	Altered state of consciousness in which the subject is open to suggestions	Treatment of illnesses and/or anesthetic treatment	Some success; further study needed
Human Cybernetics	Create receptive state of mind to accomplish healing of self	Initiate self-healing	Documentation needed
Impact Therapy	Disabled part of body is firmly supported between two bags of sand; third sand bag is raised and lowered rhymically, causing pressure waves	Reduces pain and swelling of joints	Documentation needed
Iridology	Observe condition of iris: clarity and brightness of color; shades within basic color; texture of iris; characteristics of fibers and rings used as indicators of systemic conditions	Indicates general health of the rest of the body	Condition of eyes is an indicator of some diseases, but the extensive claims of iris diagnosis are questioned; documentation needed
Kirlian Photography	Electrophotography of a body's energy aura	Predict disease or imminent death	Limited scientific evidence
Lakhovsky Oscillatory Coils	Apparatus emits electromagnetic field; and patient is placed in the field	Restores cells to healthy vibration pattern	Quackery by present standards
Luscher Color Test	Have person choose colors in order of preference	Indicates state of mind and/or glandular balance	Scientific documentation needed
Medical Radiesthesia	Diagnose disease by using pendulum over diagnostic chart with drop of patient's blood on it; deviations of pendulum indicate disease or organ affected	Diagnoses diseases; especially disease factors not easily identified by standard clinical tests	Documentation needed; considered quackery by present standards
Metaphysical Healing	Prayer to God to eliminate ill health	Healing	Documentation needed
Meditation	Learning to free mind from the known. Discover peace	Learn to know oneself; develop inner strength and peace	Documentation needed

MEDICAL THEORY, THERAPY OR APPROACH	TECHNIQUE OR PROCEDURE	BENEFIT CLAIMED	VALIDITY
Moxibustion	Herb cone is placed along meridians, burned down almost to skin, and then quickly removed; used in conjunction with acupuncture	Stimulates body's life energy	Documentation needed
Neurophysiological	View person and his problems from relationship between mind, body, behavior, and emotions. Wholistic approach	Treat emotional or stress disorders	Documentation needed
Orgone Therapy	Raise charge of blood	Combat illness	Quackery by present standards
Osteopathy	Manipulation of the body, especially the spinal column; involves rhythmic movements and massage of areas that may be causing constrictions of nerves, circulatory system, or hormonal system	Heals variety of illnesses and diseases	Recognized by some as equivalent to orthodox medicine; largest of the unorthodox medical groups
Psionic Medicine	A drop of blood is used to determine cause of imbalance and disharmony in vital dynamics causing disease	Discover what will eliminate causal factors of disease and restore balance	Quackery by present standards
Psychic Diagnosis	One person attunes his or her mind to others to make contact with inner awareness	Psychic can sense (diagnose) what is wrong with the other	Scientific documentation needed
Psychic Surgery	Surgical approach used to "disconnect body energy" from diseased organs and destroy it; violates orthodox surgery, as surgeon uses no sterilization or anesthetic	Disease treatment	Quackery by present standards

130

Pyramid Energy	Place patient in pyramid structure	Cuts, wounds, and bruises heal faster, and meditation improves	Documentation needed
Radionics	Use of Standard Delaware Diagnostic instrument; a drop of patient's blood is placed in the instrument	Diagnose and treat disease at a distance	Quackery by present standards
Radionic Photography	Energy radiations from patient's blood specimen produce image on photographic plate	Confirm diagnosis	Documentation needed
Reflexology (zone therapy)	Massage certain areas of feet	Brings body back into state of balance; imbalance causes disease	Documentation needed
Rolfing	Deep massage; manipulating body to return it to healthy postural position	As body reflects mental emotional attitudes, massage of this sort frees mind and emotions from "blocks" so subject can be aware that there is free choice of action; no longer hampered by past experiences	Documentation needed
Shiatsu Massage	Finger pressure massage of the same meridian paths or pressure points used acupuncture	Relieves pain and revitalizes patients	Oriental practice; documentation needed
Skin Brushing	Brush skin daily (skin must be dry)	Remove dead skin and open pores so wastes can escape	Documentation needed
Tongue Diagnosis	Observe general appearance of tongue	Indicates any vitamin deficiency, especially of vitamin B	Valid in some circumstances
Water Therapy (cold and hot baths, sitz and sweat baths, douches, steaming, enemas, inhalation)	Apply water to skin in various ways and take internally	Therapeutic value to various body parts; increases efficiency of sweat glands; aids in blood circulation	Accepted practices provided they are not excessive

INDEX

133